MW00736996

Flight of the Beautiful Lie:

A Memoir

Jasmine Christine Ford

Dedication

"Flight of the Beautiful Lie" is dedi-
cated to all of the strong black super-
women in my family, and those I have been
blessed enough to encounter, throughout
the course of my life. I say to you, your
love, guidance, and prayers were never
wasted. And to my dearest Alease Ford, my
great-grandmother, rest sweetly, knowing
that your great grandchild, found their
healing power after all. It was within me
all the time, just like you have always
said.

Rosalie Ford
12/24/1928 to 4/1979
maternal grandmother

Alease Ford
3/16/1907 to 4/1981
maternal great-grandmother

Carla Ford
6/11/1953 to 5/23/2013
beloved mother

Gearldine "Hattie" Overton.
9/13/1903 to 6/30/2004
maternal great-grandmother

Mary Ellen Johnson
12/24/1929 to 12/25/2009
great aunt

Ernestine Ford
8/3/1975-
beloved sister

Contents

Sin...

Sin is likened to a single
weed dwarfed in a field of
tall red roses-

Innocuous and sweet.

Obscured by the abundant
beauty about,

It matures in solitude.

Quietly among thorns
and thistles it grows in
character-

Perfecting its play, day
after day.   Until

Sin is likened to a sea of
weeds roaring around a single
wilted rose.

J.C. Ford, 2015

Introduction

The Greyhound bus came to a complete stop at the corner of Seventh Avenue and 32nd Street. I was the last passenger to step down onto the busy streets of New York. The obnoxiously bright neon lights, mixed with the sounds of car horns, music, and loud voices, made me smile broadly. I was home again. As I made my way up the avenue with my suitcase trailing behind me, the thought hit me like a ton of bricks: for the first time in 30 years, I was not in the city on business. I was here for me.

By the time I approached the revolving doors of the Hotel Pennsylvania, the paisley summer dress I was wearing had already begun to cling to the contours of my curves. I had braved a five-hour bus ride from Washington, DC in the middle of August, and I had the sweat to show for it. I didn't have time or money to actually rent a room. I fell into a chair, nervous and exhausted.

In a few hours, I would be across town at NYU Langone Medical Center, receiving a vaginoplasty — the last in a long series of surgeries I had undergone over a period of many years. (I know this is the first page of this book, and I want you to keep reading, so I'm not going to describe the operation to you in detail. But things *will* get graphic as my story goes on; definitely consider yourself warned.) I would ultimately be in the hospital for close to a week recovering from the operation. But for now, I was all alone, in a familiar city but far from home, embarking on an unfamiliar and frightening journey.

As I sat with my suitcase and my thoughts, a man came across the lobby to speak to me. "Why is a beautiful girl like you sitting down here by yourself?" he asked.

I'd heard this sappy line more times than I could count, but rarely this early in the morning. I glanced up and scanned the specimen from head to toe, like the consummate professional I had been for so many years. It's the only way to be safe and the most effective way to discern a viable trick from just another broke freak off the dirty streets of New York.

He was possibly Israeli, Middle Eastern for sure — maybe sixty years old, in decent shape with salt-and-pepper hair and kind, friendly eyes. He had on Brunello Cucinelli moccasins and a Rolex watch. Mrs. Jasmine knows her fashion. I could tell we were about the same height, and he wasn't obviously physically stronger than me. I looked around the lobby one more time; we were in a nice hotel. No obvious alarm bells were going off in my head.

"Well," I said, "I'm in town because I'm going to be checking into the hospital this morning, and I'm just down here for now, you know." I did need help, but I wasn't going to expose myself as vulnerable; I opted to be charming, as if we'd met late in the evening in the hotel bar. I repositioned myself in the leather chair I was sitting in to appear to engage him with more interest, and to give him a better view of the triple Ds that were bubblin' up at the top of my dress.

He replied, "You know what? I have a room upstairs, and you're welcome to lay on the couch until you need to leave. I promise I'm not trying to pick you up in any wrong way — you look like a nice girl who needs some help."

I told myself, *He looks harmless enough, and doesn't look stupid enough to try something with a sista anyway.*

I agreed, and followed him upstairs with my luggage.

His room was small; not a suite, but nice. I scanned the room the same way I'd scanned him. He said that his family was in the jewelry business, and that he was in New York on business. I looked around and saw expensive luggage spread out, the way a traveling businessman would treat a hotel room: comfortable, but organized well enough that nothing would get lost or left behind, and there would be no panic or rush when checkout time arrived. I felt safe, and relaxed.

I went into the bathroom to change into stretch bike shorts and the rest of my outfit. I wasn't going to undress in front of him. When I came back, we dimmed the lights and laid down on the bed. I kept my purse strap wrapped around my arm, tucking the bag itself under my head like a pillow. My suitcase was by my side. These were the tricks of my trade, learned from years of experience. As safe as I felt, I was still in a hotel room with a strange man. If things went sideways, I had to be able to leap to my feet, whip his ass, grab all of my belongings, and dash.

He didn't get close at first. We talked, and even though I was very tired after the long bus ride, I tried not to drift off to sleep because, again, I didn't know him. Still, the bed was so comfortable and so welcoming that I soon drifted in and out. He slid closer, and I let him, because he was harmless. I'd had sex for money plenty of times; I knew the game. Hell, I wrote the playbook. But I felt in my spirit that this man only wanted company. He wanted the warmth of my body. I was an attractive woman, but he didn't grope me — he put his arm around me as though we were two lovers taking a nap. I felt strangely comforted — secure — in the arms of this stranger from a foreign land.

He fell asleep before I did; his breathing steadied and grew heavier, and he barely moved. I allowed myself to sleep as well. I set my alarm for 5:30 AM, and when it went off, I got up, moving his arm aside, and went into the bathroom.

I had to do an extensive pre-surgical routine using a betadine surgical scrub that my doctor had given me. I had to focus on my perineal area, between my legs, because of the surgery I was having performed. I washed everything. After a long shower, I wiped away the condensation that had collected on the bathroom mirror, and I just stood there watching myself. My gaze traveled down my reflection and rested on my penis. In a twisted way, it appeared to be looking back at me somehow. It was limp and pitiful. "Most of you will be tucked into my vagina, and the rest will be made into my clitoris and labia, so we're not really saying goodbye," I whispered to my penis and quickly tucked it between my legs. I got dressed, and exited the bathroom with all my bags. When I came out, he was up as well, gathering himself.

He looked at me and said, "Thank you for last night. I was lonely, and you're very nice. I go all around the world and I get a good sense of who people are almost right away, and you're a nice lady." He handed me a roll of bills and said, "It's not much, but this should help you."

I could see at least two twenties on the outside when he handed it to me, but I didn't count the money. I was grateful for all the kindness he'd shown me. He kissed me on the cheek, hugged me, and I left the room. He never knew that I was transgender, that I was having a sex change that morning, or how much stress I was under the night before the biggest surgery of my life. I never said anything, and I continued on my journey by myself, and he went on his way, back to Europe or the Middle East or wherever, never knowing the impact he had on me.

Before I'd left for New York, my co-workers had thrown me a pre-operation party, with cake and everything - I knew they fully supported me and were looking forward to having me back. But I was in the city alone, and I would be spending my recovery alone. I've always gone through my toughest moments alone, and when someone has stepped up and helped, it's always seemed to be a stranger. People I don't know have been willing to offer assistance and support and even love, when members of my family or people I've been much closer to have not.

I took a taxi across town to the hospital, which was located on First Avenue, overlooking the East River. It was just before dawn, and still dark outside when I arrived. I rolled my suitcase inside, and immediately felt differently than I had during any of my other surgeries.

Surgery is always nerve-racking. You can't help but think about what's going to happen. You get all the lab work done in advance, you do all the pre-surgical work-ups with your doctor, and you're expecting to come out better, whether the procedure is to cure a disease or to make a cosmetic change. You plan for the procedure to go smoothly, and for your body to heal. I had been through it many times. But this oper-ation was different. It felt like there was something uniquely final about this last procedure.

The surgical suite was on the second floor. When I arrived, I was the only per-son in the waiting room, and it was quite cool, even cold. It was a strange feeling, almost like being in a dream about going to a hospital, especially since the facil-ity itself was very new and everything seemed to gleam. I sat by myself thinking, *I'm going to go through those double doors and I'm going to wake up forever changed.*

After a few minutes, a woman arrived to open up the surgical suite and sat behind the desk. I approached her and gave her my name and my insurance information, the whole intake procedure that was so familiar. She told me I would be escorted back within 15 or 20 minutes.

I went back to my seat, my nervousness increasing, and took ten minutes to log into Facebook and post. I shot a short video of myself, which is still on my page. I thanked all my people — the aunts who had raised me, both those who are still living and those who were dead, and everyone who was supportive of me. I did that because I truly didn't know if I was going to come out of the operation. You never know if you're going to survive surgery, so as a deeply spiritual person, I wanted to state clearly that I was okay with the Lord before anything occurred. I'm not afraid of death — not after the life I've lived — but I always want to be prepared for death. So, I made that post, and a few people saw it and chimed in.

Right after that, a nurse came and brought me through the double doors leading to the surgical suite. There was a small side room where I had to get undressed. I undressed very slowly, because this was the last time I was ever going to have this kind of body, the body I'd had for 46 years. That's a long time, and although

I may not have always wanted to have a penis, and may have abused it at times, in good and bad ways, it was mine. And in a few short hours, it wasn't going to be there anymore.

I didn't know exactly how I was going to feel about that. I was happy – this was the final stage in a process that had taken years and cost staggering amounts of money – but I was also sad about the change. I didn't know how my life would be after this procedure. I had been defined by being transgender for so long. I was a girl with a penis – a pretty girl, with a nice face and body, but a girl with a penis. That had been my identity for almost three decades. And before that, I had been a boy who wanted to be a girl. I had never been a total woman, with all the parts, but within a few hours I was going to know and feel that experience; that would be my life. It was frightening, and yes, a little sad.

The staff were as nice as I could have hoped. Once I undressed and put on the surgical gown, they came to my room and introduced themselves. They all knew why I was there, and everyone involved was 100 percent affirming. I felt affirmed as a woman, and validated as a person who was opting for a sex change. I have to say, I paid a fortune, but I felt like I got my money's worth. My insurance paid the hospital $185,000 but from the moment I walked through the doors to the moment I walked back out, they earned every penny. They treated me like a queen, and my hospital bed was my throne. I really needed that validation from an emotional standpoint. My body was bruised and swollen, but my heart was full.

My doctor, Dr. Rachel Bluebond-Langner, was the last person to come in. She has blond hair and at that time was in her late thirties, perhaps her early forties. She was immaculately dressed in a knee-length Chanel dress and what looked like Ralph Lauren loafers from his new summer arrival collection. During one of the most important moments of my life, I couldn't shake the recurring question that flooded my mind: What surgeon wears Chanel to perform surgery at seven in the morning? *My* surgeon, dammit, and she was *fabulous*.

She entered the room and immediately hugged me, asking, "Are you ready? Today is your day. You're gonna walk out of here a beautiful girl!" Hearing those words made me smile; my fears were slowly dissipating.

It was about seven AM when they put me in a wheelchair and rolled me into the operating theater. I was surprised by how crowded the room was. Everything was new — the bed, the surgical equipment, all of the computers (the procedure required lasers to measure the depth of my vagina) and the other technical equipment. I was a little bit stunned by it all, but most of all by the people. You see, Dr. Bluebond-Langner was a teaching physician, and she was showing a bunch of medical students her special technique. Several of them weren't doctors yet, while others were doing their residencies, but there were about ten people in the room besides me. They were very sweet, though — young and friendly, and eager to observe.

I laid down on a table that had extended legs with stirrup-like fittings to hold my heels, as though I was about to give birth. The nurse connected the IV to my arm and I looked around. All the strangers around me were talking with each other, looking down at their pre-operative checklists. To them it was routine, but I was about to change the course of the rest of my life. I hoped that it would be a positive outcome, but I wasn't sure — I couldn't be sure until it was over. Everyone else was free to think *Oh, it's just surgery*, but it was my body. It was my life. When they all went home for the night, I was either going to have a vagina and love it, or have a vagina and hate it, but there would be absolutely no turning back.

A flood of memories rushed through my mind – my childhood; the first time I took hormones and developed breasts, and how thrilling it was; my surgery to get breast implants; all the other operations after that…

And, of course my faith filled my mind, too. Was I making the right decision? Was God going to love the new me? I began to cry, lying there as they moved around me, putting things on my arms, and covering me with a body warmer because I had begun to shiver.

A nurse leaned over and asked, "Why are you crying?"

I said, "This is just…" and I couldn't even finish my sentence, but she understood. She laid her hands over mine, patting me softly.

"It's going to be okay, Jasmine," she said. Then she said, "I'm going to ask you to count back from one hundred down to one, and you're going to feel a warm sensation in your IV – that's to put you to sleep, and when you wake up, it'll all be over, and you'll be on your way to a new life."

When she said that, a fresh wave of tears rolled down my face. I started counting down – "Ninety-nine, ninety-eight, ninety-seven…"

By the time I got to 94, I was out.

Chapter 1: Little Boy Lost

It was negative one degrees Celsius, windy and snowing in Philadelphia, Pennsylvania on March 5th, 1972 at exactly 12:15 AM, the day I arrived into the world. I was born to a warm, smart and caring 18-year-old mother named Ester Carla Ford, who affectionately answered *only* to Carla. She named her first-born child after her own father and grandfather. My name was James Otis Ford, but I answered to the nickname Jof, which was an acronym of my full name.

The story between my mother and father was never made entirely clear to me, but what was abundantly clear was that he wasn't around, and my mother absolutely loathed the man, at least by the time I came along. My earliest and only memory of him occurred when I was about five years old. One hot summer day, I remember two nicely dressed men with significantly large hair walking up to me while I was sitting on my grandma's porch playing jacks with four other neighborhood children.

One of the men approached me as I played, patted me on the head and said, "Hey Jof!" The big-haired stranger spoke with an air of familiarity as he ran his large fingers through my coarse head of hair. I was instantly perplexed, and honestly a little scared. "Do you know who I am?" he continued. I looked up at the tall figure and slowly shook my head no. He got closer to me, squatted down to nearly my height and responded, "Well, I'm your dad, and this is your uncle…" and introduced me to the man with him. The other man, who was standing closer to the curb, walked over and extended his hand for a handshake. As I placed my hand in his, I remember he had a wide friendly smile with a slight gap between his front teeth. The encounter with my apparent father was such a brief and awkward exchange, the name of his brother, my uncle, didn't have enough time to sink into my memory. I believe it might have been John or Steven. The man who patted me on the head, and unceremoniously announced that he was in fact my father, slid a crumpled five-dollar bill into the palm of my tiny, dirty hand, and continued bopping down Cantrell Street.

Minutes later, the loud commotion of little voices, presumably over a game, brought my mother to the doorway to investigate. When she arrived, she found herself in the middle of a four-way shoving match. "Let me see the money?" skinny, snaggle-toothed LJ said.

"See with your eyes and not with your hands," I teased, waving the crinkled bill over my head like a miniature flag. Snot-nose Marvin from Winton Street, which ran parallel to Cantrell, tried to give his victim impact statement to the rest of us from the first step on the stoop. "I don't have a fadder, but if I had a fadder who gave me money I would share it with you, just like I share my ice cream my nana bought yesterday," he said, sucking snot back into his nose.

"I only took *one* lick," I snapped.

"What is going on out here?" my mother asked, apparently listening to the ruckus from the doorway. "And where did you get that money that's in your hand Jof?"

Like an unsynchronized gaggle of guppies, a porch full of five- and six-year-old kids chimed in before I could offer a single word. "A man with a big ol' afro come walking down the street and slapped Jof upside his peanut head and said that him was his fadder," Said LJ.

Somebody else continued the story with their version and said, "Yeah Mrs. Carla, and gave Jof money to buy everybody ice cream and candy and him just walked away. His father is a nice man." The second boy's name was Rudy. He was that neighborhood kid that was my age but looked two years older and was nearly 30 pounds heavier. From my observation back then, anyone who came within arm's reach of Rudy with candy, food or money to buy candy or food in his astute opinion were all nice people.

"Rip it up!" my mother yelled. "I don't know who in the hell that man was. But that man wasn't your father. Do you hear me. Do you understand me Jof? You don't have a father," she said in front of all my little playmates. "As a matter of fact, *I'm* your father. If that good for nothin' nigga ever bring his ass around here again, I want you to run and get me. You're not to go anywhere with him or anyone associated with him. You're not to even *speak* to him again. Understand?"

"Yes, mommy," I said, and ripped the crumpled bill into as many pieces as I could, to my mother's satisfaction and to Rudy's horror. What stuck out so poignantly was her bitter anger about the whole situation; it was obvious that by that time she absolutely hated my father with a passion, and to this day I don't completely understand why. That was an impression that was confirmed for me years later, when he and I met again. I never saw him again as a child — we had no relationship, he had no fatherly wisdom or life lessons to pass down — until I was 14. One day I got a phone call out of the blue, and from that point we attempted to have a relationship. That didn't last long.

When I was very young, my mother began to exhibit mental and emotional issues, and was eventually diagnosed as schizophrenic with depressive episodes. I'm not entirely sure where it came from; I've heard from some relatives that my mother abused drugs and subsequently got what's known as a "hot shot," meaning that the drugs were contaminated in some way that caused her schizophrenia. Other people say that it simply developed organically. I later come to learn through my own education that the onset of schizophrenia is first exhibited in young adults. Whatever the case may be, she was suffering a great deal, and was in and out of mental institutions and State hospitals most of my young life. Although my mother was not a constant fixture in the lives of my sister and me, her love for us was undeniable and never wavered as she weathered the storms of her mental illness and drug addiction.

I adored my mother, but life was challenging and at times confusing, because when you're a small child, you don't have a real sense of time as a linear concept of chronology. Days pass by in a blur, and you mostly remember standout experiences, like a special trip to the zoo, a birthday where you receive everything on your wish list, and yes, even a handful of confetti that was once a crumpled five-dollar bill — which incidentally turned out to be the only gift my father ever gave me.

Because of my mother's illness, I spent much of my early life living with my grandmother Roselee, my mother's mother; my Aunt Harriett, who was actually my mother's first cousin; and my great-grandmother.

Her last name was Ford, like mine, all of the old folks called her "Fordie," and everyone else referred to her respectfully as Mrs. Ford. She was the mother of my grandfather on my mother's side; I was told he died while serving in the military.

Grandma Ford was dressed in dark cocoa brown skin that still shimmered when the light reflected off of it. In her mid-seventies she had the kind of smile that made me feel warm and fuzzy on the inside. My younger sister, Ernestine Tina Ford, came along exactly three and a half years after me. Unlike me, my sister knew almost nothing about her father, not his full name, a pat on the head, nor a crumpled-up five-dollar bill. All we could ever ascertain was that he cared strongly for our mother, was at the very least biracial, and died either shortly before or after she was born on August 3rd, 1975.

When Tina was born she looked like a ray of sunshine, and she followed her older brother around the house like a little lost puppy dog, just as soon as she was able to crawl. For the first few years of her life, I was all she knew. I loved and adored my sister. She and I were a package deal and everyone in the family knew it.

Throughout our early childhood, our mother was in and out of the State Hospital, so my sister and I were partially raised by our Grandma Ford, our mother's paternal grandmother.

Grandma Ford said to me anytime we were alone, "Jof, take care of your little sister because all you have is each other, and it's gonna be that strong bond that's gonna help you two get through life in one piece." She would always drop gems of wisdom while giving us bubble baths, as we ate scrapple, grits and eggs at the breakfast table, or when tucking us into her bed after we'd said our prayers.

As an innocent child, these "speeches" were nothing more than "old folk talk" that was to be respectfully tolerated but never really understood. Grandma knew exactly what she was doing. As I reflect on how my life unfolded over many years, I am now convinced that those ominous conversations between Fordie, Tina and me foreshadowed events that would dramatically alter the trajectory of our lives. What did she know? What did the Holy Spirit whisper in her ear during those long hours they spent together in prayer?

Oh my goodness, did I have a praying great-grandmother. I would hear her up late at night asking the Lord to cover her grans and great grans in the name of Jesus. "Lord, please regulate Carla's mind and bring her back to these churn'n. Lord bless Sunny, Elise, Katrinka, Terrell, and Dondi. Lord have your way. Watch over the Fords, Pailins and Overtons. Meet them at the point of their need o Lord in Jesus name…" I would often drift off to sleep in her bed to the sound of whispered prayers, and awaken to see her in the same position the following morning: hands folded, eyes closed, sitting in her favorite chair in front of the mahogany dresser in her bed-room. She would rise with the sun for her morning prayer.

Grandma would often lay hands on her-self for deliverance from the excruciat-ing pain that her rheumatoid arthritis and fibromyalgia brought her practically every minute of her day. She believed in her God for any and everything. The old lady knew from walking with the Lord all of her life that "…the effectual fervent prayer of the righteous availeth much." Unbeknownst to me at the time, I was and still am the recip-ient of the fruit of her fervent prayers (keep reading, the evidence will speak for itself).

The inner strength, faith and fortitude of that old woman God sent to be my great-grandmother was my earliest example of a superwoman. I am blessed enough to have had five in my lifetime thus far. It moves me to tears even while writing these words, that Grandma Ford prayed for me in pain, covered my ailing body in salves and ointment while her own body was racked with pain, and slaved over a hot stove many a day while arthritic hands struggled to manipulate cast iron pots and pans to keep our bellies from mashing against our backbones. Her failing knees would meet the creaking wooden floor each night to fellowship with the God she loved more than anything in this world.

The fondest memory I have of Grandma Ford was serving as her chief helper, or so she would call me. We lived in a row house in the five hundred block of Cantrell Street in South Philadelphia. Everyone who is familiar with Philly is aware of a few undisputable facts: Philadelphia is the home of the best cheesesteaks bar none, has the narrowest side streets in the entire northeast region of the country, and the stairs in old row homes are steep as hell. While living with my grandma I was only responsible for two things: being a good boy, and to help Gran climb those steep-ass stairs come nightfall.

"Come on baby, it's time for bed. Turn the television off and grab my purse next to my chair. Do like you always do and help great-grandma up the stairs," she'd say as she slowly got up from her favorite chair in the front room.

"Yes, Grandma," I replied and sprang to my feet. We had a rhythm to our nightly ritual. With her walking cane in my left hand and her purse dangling from my right shoulder, we were off. I would climb the first five steps or so ahead of her, care-fully turn around with everything I was lugging and would sit on that fifth step facing her. I knew that the first step was the most painful, so I would always give her an encouraging smile as I sat waiting above.

Her ascension to her bedroom every night invariably started and ended the same way; with a grimace on her face and a deep grunt through tightly pursed lips. And then sec-onds later, it started. "Oh Lord, give me strength to get up these stairs." She cried out to God as her voice cracked and shook from the pain radiating from her weak, deteriorating knees. Years of rheumatoid arthritis had left her articulating knee joints grating bone against bone with very little lubricating fluid.

"That's it, Grandma. You're almost to me." I said, as I scooted backwards up a few more steps.

"Jesus!" She begged in agony as she braved the eighth step. Tiny beads of sweat moistened her brow. Slightly deformed hands, the result of illness and age, gripped the banister and pulled. She was almost there. I was now at the top of the staircase, looking down. Our eyes locked and she blurted out her very last prayer. "Lord Almighty! Help me get to this child, Father. I'm all he's got." And just like that, the Lord granted her the last step. She made it. She always did.

Unbeknownst to me, there would come a time very soon when the first superwoman I've ever known would be defeated by her flesh, unable to rescue the little boy she so dearly loved, who patiently waited, night after night, at the top of the stairs. But that night when Grandma reached the top of the stairs, she wrapped those

ailing hands around me and we both cele-
brated in laughter. Grandma would laugh so
hard that her big brown eyes would disap-
pear behind two slits with deep wrinkles
around them. In between, while catching
a breath, she exclaimed, "Ain't God good
baby? He's so good. The Good Lord put you
here for a reason. Yes siree!" She cut her
smile off sharply and just stared at me
for a few seconds as though she could see
straight through me. "Those who love the
Lord are gifted with spiritual gifts, and
your spiritual gift is that of a healer
and encourager, I believe. As a matter of
fact, I just know it."

I grinned a shy grin, threw my head
back and laughed. It tickled me deeply
just to imagine that the almight God, cre-
ator of all things, thought me special
enough to bestow gifts and talents to me,
in order to be of service to others. "I'm
a healer, Grandma?" I asked as I crawled
into her bed.

"Yes Jof, you're a healer," she replied,
as she ran her hand gently over my head.

I conjured up my healing power as I
rooted my body underneath the covers. "In
Jesus name I heal my mommy, my grandma,
my great grandma..." I rattled off a few

more names of people I wanted to heal as I dozed off to sleep.

I had an ordinary 1970s inner-city childhood. I dressed like any other kid from South Philly during that era — bell bottom corduroy slacks, multi-colored crew neck tops and tennis shoes. Although my mother had many personal challenges when I was a young child in her care, she saw to it that my baby sister and I were always clean and well dressed. And if our mother did drop the ball because of her mental illness, her mother, Rosalee, was only too willing to pick up where her daughter left off concerning her grandchildren.

I have a keen memory of loving to dance, no matter what may have been going on around me. I remember the joy of twirling around my great-grandmother's house and grooving to the hippest tunes played on the television show *Soul Train*. In those days *Soul Train* was a relatively new entertainment show that quickly became the cat's meow. Tina and I would sometimes put on a show during the program for our mother, grandmother, uncle or whoever was at the house at that time. We would join in as Ike and Tina shook a tail feather, James Brown gyrated like a "Sex Machine," whatever that was, and mother never needed a reason to belt out the lyrics to Earth, Wind and Fire's song "Reason."

It was during times like these when our mother appeared to us to be "normal," for lack of a better word. I can recall times when our mother was emotionally present, kind, funny, creative and patient, and then there were times when she would vacillate sharply from having a flat affect (unable to ascertain what an individual was thinking or feeling due to their lack of physical cues) to displaying a cascade of emotions, sometimes in a relatively short period of time. I am not sure of the timetable, but eventually Mother began to not just hear voices, and have complete conversations with individuals and in some instances "beings" that weren't there, she would draw my sister and me into her vivid hallucinations.

I never thought as a child that my mother was mentally ill. I internalized her personality as being incredibly creative during playtime, and persistently tired or despondent at other times, and I believed it was my perpetual job to cheer her up. My life as a child was akin to a balancing act, where I constantly walked on eggshells when my mother was around. I never knew which version of her my sister and I would get from day to day — sometimes hour to hour. That was our life. When she became really ill, my mother would either check herself into the hospital for psychiatric care or be encouraged to seek treatment from various family members.

Something definitely happened at the age of six. One day it occurred to me in a very peculiar way that I paid far more attention to little boys than girls. Not just paid more attention to, but I desired their approval. I desired their approval the way grown-up boys fluttered around grown-up girls like lost puppy dogs, hungrily nibbling at scraps of validation rendered from long, delicate, perfumed fingers. I realize that imagery is rather mature for a child, but that was what I wanted — or some semblance of that. And I became eager to express myself more and more.

There was a very large vacant lot in the middle of my grandmother's block that separated Cantrell from Winton Street, where homes had been either burned down or demolished. Trees and overgrown weeds now occupied the space. Every day when the weather was nice, I would trek across that urban jungle to play with friends who lived in the neighboring block. I often played with the Evans boys and their cousins. We played games like hopscotch, kickball, stickball hide and seek, kiss-and-run and my favorite – house. (What can I say? We were a bunch of "fast ass" little kids.)

Hopscotch was a game that we played either on the sidewalk or in the street, kickball and stickball were played in a dirt clearing in the vacant lot and house was quietly played in the basement of the Evans' home. Before we even hit the bottom step of the basement, I would have already called mother. Kevin Evans always wanted to be the father. "Why do you always gotta be the mother or daughter? You're a *boy*, Jof!" Little Stephanie said.

"I can be a girl for play if I want to," I snapped. "And besides, you don't make the rules. The boys make the rules." I turned to Kevin with my hands on my hip. "Who do you want to be the mother Kevin, me or Stephanie?" I demanded.

"Well Jof, you always play my wife, so why don't we let Stephanie get a turn?" Kevin said diplomatically as he stared at the concrete floor. He knew what was coming.

"I'm leaving!" I blurted as I slammed down the toys that I was playing with and raced up the stairs.

"Where are you going?" he yelled.

"I'm going home. I quit," I yelled back. Kevin walked to the base of the stairs and looked up at me. He was brown-skin with brownish-green eyes that twinkled in the sunlight. He smiled at me apologetically.

Kevin had a dimple in the middle of his chin like white men did in old cowboy-and-Indian movies. His bright smile always gave me junior butterflies, but I had to stand my ground in front of that heifer Stephanie.

"How about you be the daughter?" I cut my eyes over at her. I never remember seeing a seven-year-old look so damn smug and satisfied in my entire young life. Stephanie was admittedly a striking golden-brown complected little girl, with coffee colored kinky textured hair that lightly dusted the middle of her back. She had big dough eyes like Bambi that she would roll and swim, either in disgust or approval at a whim. Everyone made a fuss over Stephanie, especially the adults. To put it frankly, if beauty pageants was a "thing" for little black girls in South Philly in 1979,

I imagined that Stephanie would have had a pink bedroom lined with trophies and accolades. But in my biased opinion, she was nothing short of an overrated, ghetto-fied, bargain basement beauty, who by the Grace of God, squawked when she sang. I envied her. I literally wanted to scratch her face raw.

"What, Kevin? Be the daughter, so you two can send me to bed...alone? No thank you." I was jealous, mortified and leaving. "And you better tell your fat ugly brother Michael to give me back *all* of my G.I. Joe men, and they better not have cooties on them either." I said as I slammed his front door. Play dates like the one I just described were not typical; however, mathematically speaking, friendship plus competition will always equal contention at some point. And kids will be kids regardless of the generation they happen to have been born in.

At the end of those fun, albeit contentious days, when the sun went down and the streetlights came on, I would have to cross that dark vacant lot to get home. During the day it served as the neatest backdrop to some of the coolest games and adventures, but at night the lot became one of the most dangerous areas in the neighborhood. Under the cover of darkness, drug addicts would use some of the decimated structures as safe havens to either score or use, while the neighborhood loose booty (the equivalent of your garden variety early twenty-first century "thot") commenced to doing her civic duty by performing various sex acts with random men from the neighborhood simply for shits and giggles, and where, according to my mother, faggots would run trains on each other on old dirty, pissy, discarded mattresses. The scene was exactly what a lot of suburban whites would refer to as "the ghetto."

My mother's brother Uncle Sunny or my mother would stand on my grandmother's stoop and call out to me from across the lot when it was time for me to come in for the night. "Jof, come on home. It's almost dark," my mother would say. I almost never stopped playing when she first shouted out to me.

"Okay, mom!" I'd yell back from across the dusty lot. "Another ten minutes, mom," I said back.

Thirty minutes later the whole block heard, "Jof, bring your black ass in this house right now." I immediately dropped whatever I was doing and headed toward the dark lot. As I approached, I heard my mother's voice and saw her standing on the stoop in the distance. "I can see you. Take your time. Run. Don't stop to touch anything." My mother's somewhat confusing instructions safely navigated me home.

When I was seven-and-a-half years old, my great-great-uncle Leo Pailin passed away. Uncle Leo was the brother of my great grandmother, whom everyone referred to fondly as Momma Gearl. He resided in the seven hundred block of Winton Street, across from his brother Uncle Nathan and his family. When I was a kid living in South Philly, it was common to run into family members distant or close in my old neigh-borhood, especially between the streets of 5th and 10th.

By the time my Uncle Leo passed away, the family had already suffered a great deal of tragedy and death. Our mother was once again in a psychiatric facility and hadn't been home in quite some time, her mother, grandma Rosalee had also gone home to be with the Lord, and Great Grandma Ford had suffered a heart attack and wasn't doing well in the hospital. My sister and I remember vividly during this period in our lives how we literally bounced around from family member to family member. We bounced around South Philadelphia analogous to the round silver metal object striking feverishly against taunt rubber bands scattered about in an old pinball machine-fast and furious. If the uncertainty of where we were going to lay our head down at night as children wasn't emotionally destabilizing enough, to my chagrin, the human language spat out a pejorative phrase that described what was happening to us. The term "Pillar to post" was sometimes uttered loudly in passionate defense of our circumstance, as well as, whispered softly among gossiping adults in reference to Carla's fatherless and often times, motherless children. I was obviously too young at the time to understand the clinical implications surrounding mental illness, drug addiction, or even the financial burden associated with trying to rescue an orphaned child, but I was intimately acquainted with shame, sadness and loss by the time I was seven years old. By the time of Uncle Leo's funeral repast, and the events that occurred not because of, but as a result of his passing, only made my feelings of shame, sadness and loss more salient.

On the day of the funeral, Tina and I was being cared for by our Uncle Sunny in our Great Grandmother's house. Tina and I were no longer as well dressed or well -groomed as we once were. Uncle Sunny loved us, but he certainly wasn't winning any father of the year awards any time soon-nor any Uncle of the year awards for that matter. In hindsight I believe he did the best he could with what was available to him at that point in time; mind, body and spirit. As an aside, I later found out in my early teens during a personal conversation with my Uncle, that he himself was battling with his own addictions and demons that stemmed from unresolved issues with his sexuality, and simply didn't have the capacity to care for two small children-"even if ya'll did belong to my sick baby sister. I just couldn't do it Jof. I didn't want that level of responsibility and didn't want to have my life interrupted like that. And God knows you and Tina were better off" he confessed.

Uncle Sunny and I walked from 5th and Cantrell to 7th Street to get to Uncle Leo's house for the repast. I remember being self-conscious about the heel of my feet that kept flopping out of my shoes all the way up the block because they were an entire size too big, and the suit I was put in swallowed my small skinny frame whole- but at least I was clean. I recall that much. I had gotten a fresh haircut the day before. "Will Tina be at Uncle Leo's Uncle Sunny?" I asked as I shuffled behind him, trying my best to simultane-ously keep up with his stride and keep my shoes from flying off my feet and into the street. "Yes, cousin Stella is bringing her in a bit. Her daughter Jackie is fin-ishing up your sister's hair." From a dis-tance away, I could see a miniature crowd of people in their Sunday's best walking up and down the slender street with plates of food, drifting between Uncle Nathan's and Uncle Leo's homes. Uncle Nathan was the brother of Uncle Leo, who just passed away, and they both were the brothers of my Great Grandmother who everyone called Mommma Gearl. As I came onto the block, I remember giving hugs and kisses to what seemed to be an endless array of family members consisting of, but not limited to; Aunts, Great Aunts, Uncles, Great Uncles, 1st,2nd, 3rd and 4th cousins and dear fam-ily friends and their friends.

I saw my sister playing in the street with other kids-her hair was freshly braided but her clothes were ill-fitted and soiled. We both locked eyes. And then she tore off. She practically broke her neck running through the crowd to get to her big brother. "Joffy" she giggled. "I was waiting for you." She wrapped her hands around my neck and planted a big ol' raspberry kiss on my check. My sister was four and a half years old at the time and had the warmest disposition that would melt the heart of any and everyone who laid eyes on her. She was Shirley Temple cute- dimples included. Many members of my family on my mother's side including my sister and Uncle Sunny were considered, in the African American vernacular of the time, to be "high Yellow"(or high Yalla for black folks who originate south of the Mason-Dixon Line). Simply stated, they were very fair complected. And because my sister was so fair complected, dirt and grime had nowhere to hide on her face. She had dirt on her nose, checks and chin. Tina was the kind of little girl who loved getting dirty. "Tina what have you been doing? And why are you so dirty?" Uncle Sunny said to her as he walked up behind me. "Have ya'll seen Momma

Gearl yet? Everyone wants to see you both, Aunt Mary from Bethlehem, Aunt Desiree, Aunt Narcis. Come follow me to Uncle Leo's house. Hurry up ya'll. Today of all days, Tina you're gonna roll around in the dirt. Wow! Momma Gearl is gonna have something smart to say about the way ya'll look. Lord I just know it" Uncle Sunny said as we reached Uncle Leo's doorsteps.

In all honesty, Tina and I both stood out like a sore thumb among all of our appropriately dressed family members who attended the funeral. Tina donned a tee shirt with some sort of print on it, a pair of dirty floral print shorts, and a pair of white tennis shoes with socks, that were both now a dingy shade of dark grey. So yes, I understood my Uncle's trepidation about presenting us to his mother's mother-the matriarch of our family. And yes, she's about to let his dizzy ass have it, "and I'm just gonna stand back and see what the walls gonna look like." I slid the prior quote in retrospectively for its impact. The movie 'The Color Purple' was released almost 3 years later and became a blockbuster sensation in 1982. Celie was a beautifully tragic character that in my adulthood, I often reference.

Uncle Sunny, my sister Tina and I enter the home of Uncle Leo. The front door opened directly into the living space, and boy was the house crowded straight back to the kitchen. I don't remember exactly who were all present or where they were sitting in relation to Momma Gearl after 40 years, but I'm gonna give it a whirl. Here it goes. Sitting in the livingroom to the right of Momma Gearl were her two daughters Aunt Desiree and Aunt Narciss. Sitting immediately to her left was her daughter-in-law Aunt Mary, Aunt Mary's niece Katherine. Uncle Nathan, Momma Gearl's brother, was standing, and next to him was Uncle Frederick, Momma Gearl's son and the legal husband of Aunt Mary. Everyone called Uncle Frederick "Booster", most likely on account of how he drank like a fish. And Who incidentally, was already well on his way to getting wasted at his Uncle's repast. Everybody else slowly became background noise as the conversation turned to Tina and me.

"Sunny bring those children over here so I can see them" Momma Gearl said. Momma Gearl was sitting at the dining room table with the chairs all facing the living room. She was a light-skin petite woman who stood no more than five feet tall. She had silver framed glass, with silver hair to match. She wore a 1970's loosely quaffed pageboy haircut, a classic black sheath dress and tiered pearls. As a Great Grandmother in her mid-seventies, she was beautiful. I walked over and gave her a hug and a kiss first, and my sister followed and did the same. Momma Gearl grabbed me by my hand and slowly spun me around. I was being examined from head to toe while the whole room looked on. You could hear a mouse pissin' on cotton-it was just that quiet. "Come her Tina sweetie" Momma Gearl said. Tina took the initiative and started to spin without even being asked. She stuck her tongue out to me as she did so. "Lookie here Miss Lady, how are you gonna be as cute as a button, and as dirty as a pig in a pigpen all at the same time?" Momma Gearl said playfully. "I don't know Grandma, I just am" Tina said with her hand in her mouth. Every adult within the sound of her voice melted like cheap cheese at room temperature. That little girl could work a crowd- even looking and smelling like orphan Annie. That was talent. Grandma Gearl gave us both a big smile and asked us to sit down for a spell. Everyone's eyes fell on Momma Gearl as she slowly sat back in her chair without uttering a single word. She took a long lingering sip of tea that she grabbed from off of the dining the table behind her. You could hear a pin drop… and then IT happened.

"Sunny come over here" Momma Gearl said sternly as she sat the tea cup back on the table behind her. "Yes, Momma Gearl" he answered. "Do me a favor and just look at your sister's kids. Stand up children" she said. Tina and I stood up in the middle of the room. "It's a shame before God that these children are living the way they are in this family. "Momma Ge" Uncle Sunny began. "Shut the hell up nigga. Your mother Rosalee is turning over in her fucking grave right now because of how her grandchildren are being treated Sunny. These poor kids have been shuffled from Pillar to post, staying with this one and that one, ever since Rosalee died and Fordie caught sick. As God is my secret judge, if I wasn't an old woman, I would take Jof and Tina both and raise them myself and wouldn't ask any of you muthafuckas for a gotdamn thing. If most everyone in this room doesn't own their own home, I'm as cuckoo as a cuckoo clock, and these kids are running around Philadelphia dirty like their crazy or something" Grandma yelled. "Mother, it's not gonna make a bit of difference, if you have a heart attack behind this crazy bullshit" Uncle Booster said. "Momma Gearl I'm doing my best. Harriet and Stella help me out. I know my mother would be devastated, but I'm in no position to take care of Jof and Tina the way they should be" Uncle Sunny said. "Sunny you ain't doing a damn thing except gettin' high and having all kinds of freaks up in Fordie's house while she's in the hospital. Do you really think these corn bread fed niggas don't be putting all of your nasty ass business out in the streets Sunny? These kids don't have any business with you trying to raise them no way" Grandma said. "Mother, you know I don't usually get involved with family issues, but I wanted to take Tina home with me to Bethlehem at Rosalee's funeral, but everybody claimed she would be well taken care of, so I didn't press the matter" Aunt Mary said. "Yes, you sure did Mary" Momma Gearl said. "Harriet claimed she wanted Tina, and did a whole song and dance about not wanting her to leave Philadelphia. And look what's become of her. She looks like a damn ragamuffin" she continued. "Listen Mother Harriet ain't got no damn business trying to raise my dead sister's grandkids, because Harriet can't take care of herself. Harriet can't raise her own child. I'm raising Tony" Aunt Desiree said. "Well if the family doesn't object, Tina can come home with me to Bethlehem tonight. I already spoke to my son Jerome about Tina when I saw her running up and down the street with nobody watching her" Aunt Mary said.

"Well what about Jof Aunt Mary?" Uncle Sunny asked. "I can't take them both Momma Gearl. Tina is a little girl who need more guidance and supervision than a little boy. Besides Mother, you know I got sugar and high blood pressure" Aunt Mary replied. "You're right Mary. So much can go wrong with a liitle girl. "Well it's settled, my daughter-in-law is taking Tina to Bethlehem. Praise the Lord. Thank you Mary" Momma Gearl said. "Sunny run home and bring me everything that belongs to that child. Now listen carefully to your Aunt Mary, if it is ripped or torn, keep it. If it is old and discolored, don't pack it. If it is several sizes too big, don't bring it. Do you understand what I'm saying? Aunt Mary said. "Yes Aunt Mary, I understand" Uncle Sunny replied.

Later that evening, my sister Tina left in a vehicle with Aunt Mary, her son and her two nieces. It was the hardest thing the adults in the room could ever ask of a child, and that was to stand helplessly by while your only sibling is literally ripped from your life.

I didn't have to stay with Uncle Sunny long after that night, but my circumstances didn't improve as much as Tina's did...at least, not right away. My great Aunt Desiree lamented, and agreed to take me in. Was her motive for intervening on my behalf out of pity or a strained sense of obligation to the beloved sister she had lost? Who knows? I dare never to pose that question to her when she was alive, nor will I conjure up assumptions or cast unsubstantiated aspersions as it relates to my Aunt's motives. But after many years of turning the events of my early childhood over and over in my mind, I am comfortable in my decision to not give a damn one way or another. I will allow the consumer of my experiences to draw their own conclusions.

Just a few days after the funeral, I also packed up everything I owned that wasn't too big or tattered and journeyed to 32nd and Wharton Street in Southwest Philadelphia. Although I believe my Aunt cared for me in her own furtive way, she was not the doting nurturing kind, who clung to every adorable word uttered out of the mouth of a child. Not on your life. Aunt Desiree was an irreverent, fiery tongued grandmother in her mid-fifties, who was a bit on the surly side. With every meal she prepared for me, she served up a healthy heaping of," Jof, I can't do this shit much longer" she'd say. Or, "Sunny needs to get his muthaf**in shit together" and of course my shady favorite, even to this day, "I wouldn't take care of you if they gave me all the government assistance in the world". In short, it was pretty crystal-clear right from the beginning, the sooner someone took me off her hands, the better.

One would imagine that an eight year old child would feel terribly hurt by the awful things I've heard, but sadly, I became quite used to people informing me over and over in some form or fashion how unwanted I was. I had in some way worn out my welcome. In hindsight, based on how I later formed connections with people as an adult, I internalized that narrative projected onto me by the adults around me. As an adult, I still feel like an outsider in my own family- a realization I have accepted long ago as an unfortunate casualty of my transition. Subconsciously I believe I have purchased pseudo-friendships in my adulthood for my own comfort and convenience if I am to be honest. Based on my past experiences, I adopted a strange philosophy that, if I paid for people to hang out with me by offering to pay for everything, when I became disinterested, It would be well within my moral rights to severe the relationship at will. It was mutually beneficial. It may be hard to believe but I have even paid individuals to leave my life. It took a lot of prayers, trials and tribulations to get where I am today- an author. Keep reading, you've only scratched the surface.

Tina would call me on the phone almost every day from Aunt Mary's. She missed me terribly, and I missed her. We'd laugh and talk about everything. In Philadelphia, we had always been together; I was her big brother and guided her around the neighborhood, playing with her and keeping her by my side. Being apart felt awful for both of us.

That fall, as Thanksgiving approached, my sister called and asked if I would be coming to see her for the holiday. Aunt Mary said to Aunt Desiree, her sister-in-law, "I would really like it if Jof could come up to see Tina for Thanksgiving, because she's been calling out for her brother since she left Philadelphia. She doesn't sleep well, all she talks about is her big brother, so we have to reunite them at least for a few days to celebrate the holiday."

Aunt Desiree put me on the phone and Aunt Mary asked me, "Would you like to come to Bethlehem?" That was exactly how she asked the question; no mention was made of a short visit, or any kind of time limit.

I said instantly, "Yes, it sounds really nice, I'll be a good boy, I would love to come." In the excitement of the moment, I thought she'd invited me to live with her and Tina. I didn't understand that it was only intended to be a visit. I began whooping and hollering and jumping up and down, so excited that my Aunt Mary was taking me to Bethlehem and that I had heard it was so nice, and on and on.

When Aunt Desiree heard this, she grabbed the phone away from me and said, "Oh my God, Mary, you're taking this boy off my hands, thank you Jesus! Ain't God good? He can't stay here, I can't do it anymore Mary; I'll pack his stuff by tomorrow. When are you coming to get him? As a matter of fact, me and mother will bring him to you." She could not have been more excited to get me out of her house. As they spoke, I danced in front of the mirror in the living room that ran the entire length of the house from floor to ceiling. I did a jig from the front door to the kitchen and back. I then somehow conjured up an old Mahalia Jackson negro spiritual I'd heard Grandma Ford sing a time or two from the pit of my spirit - "Nobody knows the trouble I've seen, nobody knows my sorrow." Oh yes, ma'am! The praise was real. I was Bethlehem bound. Won't He do it?

Aunt Mary heard all of this – the excitement in my voice and the relief in Desiree's – and said to herself, *Well, I guess this is what's happening.* She later confessed that she didn't have the heart to let me down. She said to Desiree, "You know what? Just bring him. Pack up all his clothes, bring him for Thanksgiving, and he can stay."

Aunt Desiree was so happy, the first thing she did after hanging up with Mary was to call my great-grandmother who literally lived across the street. "Oh my God, Mother," she told her, "Mary is a gift from God. She's gonna take this boy, she's gonna have both of my sister's grandkids." It was very clear to me that everyone had loved my grandmother. She had been a wonderful person, and had it not been for her, my life may have had a different outcome.

Before I left, Aunt Desiree cheerfully took me shopping at Strawbridge & Clothier in Center City. She and I took the city bus. It was one of the best times I have ever had with my aunt. Come to think of it, she was the happiest I had ever seen her as well. She got me some underwear, some T-shirts, a few pairs of pants for school, two pullover sweaters, a couple of button-down shirts and a brand new suitcase to carry my new wardrobe in. The next day, Aunt Desiree and her mother, my great-grandmother, took me to Bethlehem.

I remember the Greyhound bus ride from Philadelphia to Bethlehem, Pennsylvania as vividly as though I took that trip yesterday. The date was November 26, 1980, the day before Thanksgiving. It was a cold but clear day as we made our way downtown to the Greyhound bus terminal. I was so excited to be among all of the holiday travelers, especially since I had never traveled outside of Philadelphia that I could recollect.

"Jof, you didn't leave anything at the house, did you?" Aunt Desiree asked.

"No, ma'am. I got everything," I said. I knew I had everything because she'd asked that same question while I was packing my belongings earlier that morning, again while waiting for the taxicab to pull up onto 32nd and Wharton Street to take us downtown, and once more while the three of us sat in the waiting area at the bus station. My dear aunt was many things, but subtle she was not.

I had just taken the last bite of my cheese hotdog when I heard over the intercom, "Allentown, Bethlehem, Easton and Quakertown now boarding on Terminal 10". Aunt Desiree, Grandma and I scurried to Terminal 10 right before the conductor made his announcement for the last time. "All aboard for Allentown, Bethlehem, Easton and Q u a k e r t o w n".

The seats were velvety and plush and the bus had a bathroom in the rear. Grandma let me sit by myself right across the aisle from where they sat. Oh, I was big timin'. My nose was pressed hard against the cold window of the bus as I watched the high neon PSFS sign at the top of the Philadelphia Saving Fund Society fade in the distance. And just like that, the only home I'd ever known was out of sight. Center City Philadelphia was gone.

As the Greyhound bus began its decent into Bethlehem, high on South Mountain, I got my first glimpse of the majestic Star of Bethlehem that seemingly appeared to magically hover over the mountaintop like one of God's angelic heavenly hosts. If I had any reservation or fear about moving to Bethlehem buried down deep in the recesses of my little heart, it melted away as we turned onto West 4th St. Old fashioned light poles were individually adorned with miniature Christmas trees, each one professionally trimmed with all of the bells and whistles of the festive season.

As I think about that day, there was something indescribable lingering in the air of Bethlehem that enveloped me. So much more than snowcapped mountains, a huge steel supported star planted in a clearing giving the illusion that it dangled in the evening sky, and more than millions of blinking white Christmas lights that brought the city of Bethlehem to life every night. I felt far more than my carnal senses could absorb and process. That initial indescribable feeling I later came to recognize as the overwhelming sensation one experiences when one returns home after a long arduous journey. The lost little boy I was for a very long time had found a home.

A Child's Prayer

Lord, I don't ever want to be,
too high to soar,
too lucky to learn,
too pretty to pray, or
unconcerned if you stay.

I don't ever want to be,
too big for my britches,
too arrogant for a wish list,
too useless to be used,
with a huge ego to bruise.

I don't ever want to be,
too quick to anger,
too slow to soothe,
too reticent to repent, or
deny the Son sent!

Amen...

Chapter 2: Bethlehem

Section 1 (Good Ol' Aunt Mary)

The taxicab parked near the corner of Main and Union Boulevard. My Aunt Mary lived in a big nine-room house on the north side of Bethlehem, nestled in what was referred to as the Lehigh Valley. She owned two row homes four blocks away and down the hill from the beautiful, sprawling campus of Moravian College, a private liberal arts school founded in 1742 by Moravians, where she also worked as a member of the cleaning crew.

I would spend a great deal of my childhood playing with new friends on the expansive fields that surrounded the sixth-oldest college in the country. My new schoolmates would be mostly white early on, ambitious for their age and far more privileged than the friends I left behind in South Philly. And those facts in and of themselves would later prove to be academically beneficial, socially isolating and sexually stigmatizing during crucial stages of my development. But I'm jumping ahead of myself a bit. Let me back up.

When we got within inches of the front door with our luggage in hand, Aunt Desiree turned to Momma Gearl and whispered with a smirk, "You know what's going on in there, don't you, Mother?"

"Uh huh, she in there carrying on. Got the whole house and sidewalk just a-stankin'. Now you know Mary ought to be ashamed of herself, doin' these white folks around here like this," Grandma said as she knocked three times on the beige wooden door with the large glass cut out. "Come open the door for your mother, it's cold out here, Mary."

And stankin' it certainly was, but in the best way imaginable. As soon as the three of us got out of the cab and stepped onto the sidewalk, we immediately caught a waft of fresh collard greens simmering slowly on a bed of fried salted pork slices, homemade sweet potato pie lightly dusted with powdered cinnamon, golden baked ham drizzled with glazed brown sugar bubblin' in the oven right about 365 degrees, cabbage with chunks of ham hocks, a tray of southern fried chicken (the first batch), four-cheese baked macaroni and a couple of moist, fluffy lemon pound cakes showered with freshly squeezed lemon and confection sugar. I couldn't see the ingredients my Aunt Mary used. I'm not clairvoyant. However, over the many years I would spend growing up in Bethlehem, a lot of time was spent in the kitchen with its large bay window that seeped in cold air in the winter and roasted us alive in the summer.

Aunt Mary emerged from the kitchen and opened the front door. There was chatter, smiles and hugs as we were ushered into the house through a living room area where antique furniture was encased in plastic, a more modern lived-in television room, and into the kitchen in the rear of the house, where all of the soul food magic took place. Aunt Mary was a relatively tall woman in her late fifties with a solid build, wavy salt-and-pepper hair that would have hung to the middle of her back, though she always wore it in a bun held up by a single jeweled comb.

I gazed around the kitchen at the enormous amount of food either already made or prepped and into the television room directly behind me. I was taking everything in: the sights, sounds and smells of my new home. My eyes rested on an old black-and-white photo of Aunt Mary in her youth. She wore a fur wrap and what looked like a grey pantsuit. Her hair was not fashioned like an afterthought, swirled into a bun, but fell in rich black curls down the right side of her shoulder and rested on her lapel. Not a hair out of place. She was reminiscent of old black Hollywood, a Dorothy Dandridge/Lena Horne caliber black beauty with real style. Her smiling face bore not a single blemish or flaw. The photo had me gobsmacked, and so proud to call the lady in it my aunt.

At my aunt's feet, metaphorically speaking, I'd learn of her history as a Black-Indian American with almost no formal education who grew up in a sturdy shack in Augusta, Georgia. Who would eventually work as a cook and housekeeper in order to feed her family and ultimately become a homeowner and landlord of multiple properties.

What probably impressed me the most was that the very same individual who used to cram the importance of education down the throats of the children she'd raise, or in her words, "makin' sure her churn'n get their lessons," was unable to read herself. Aunt Mary was only able to write her full name in cursive and in print. But that detail never shamed her, nor kept her from maximizing the opportunities that presented themselves throughout the course of her life, like it would have for so many others.

Education was an important commodity to her, because I suppose it represented the ultimate "power," in that whoever possessed it also possessed the ability to broker any aspect of the American dream that was lavished on so many, and denied to so many others as a consequence of intrinsic racism. My aunt shared stories of how she and others she knew struggled through and survived debilitating forms of racial injustice when she was a child. An era when the ethos of Jim Crow and the not-so-distant horror of slavery were woven into the delicate fabric of this country, and thus directly influencing the psychosocial, psychosexual, political and economic behavior of black people for generations.

In hindsight, as a middle-aged woman of color who has transitioned, I understand my aunt's strong reaction to homosexuality, especially how it directly affected her great nephew she had obligated herself to raise. She was terribly afraid for me. Afraid that the world would chew me up and spit me out, or that its perpetual cruelty would render me ineffective and inept. Obviously, I'm just surmising based on our relationship, and utilizing language most comfortable for me. However, fear about my sexuality was evident in her countenance and parenting and peaked in my preteens.

She had an idea when I was relatively young, based on my mannerisms and interests, that one day she would have to release an eighteen-year-old black male who would identify as homosexual, and who had a mild to moderate stutter, into a bigoted world. I believe that is the reason why Aunt Mary never coddled me as a child. Instead, she prepared me for life, imparting valuable life lessons that would help me develop the survival skills I would surely need once I left home. While her reaction to my budding sexuality in my youth was psychologically harmful and traumatizing at times, at other times her maturity, wisdom and acceptance shocked the hell out of me. During this chapter I will share a few interesting examples of both. But first, allow me to draw from my experiences as an adult, and provide an anecdote from my past that will put the relationship I had with my aunt in its proper context.

I was a faithful member of New Birth Baptist Church Cathedral of Faith International in Opa-locka, a city in Miami-Dade County, Florida in 2014. My group of church friends, who consisted of Renee, Raquel, Mrs. Zee, Sir Diego, Cedric Vaughn, Quinn-Quinn and myself, called ourselves "the clan." We were a band of misfits and strangelings, some would say. I came in contact with an African-American male in his mid-forties, whose name I will not reveal, but he was in town from Jacksonville, receiving treatment for crack and crystal meth addiction at an inpatient facility close to downtown. He referred to New Birth as his home away from home. Every Sunday, this gentleman would be at the second worship service, praising his heart out. He would always come alone, so the clan embraced him, and began to invite him to the many after-church outings we had at local eateries every Sunday afternoon.

When I declare that this man knew the unadulterated word of God, I mean what I say. He had the ability to recite chapter and verse verbatim. If you had a problem, concern, or question about any biblical precept, this individual could pick up a Bible and show you where in God's word where you could find resolution and clarity to any situation you were faced with. This brother walked up in church like he was a senior pastor and just as well dressed. In the words of my Aunt Mary, the brother was "shitty sharp," pardon my French. I had to know this individual's testimony.

During dinner after worship services on Thanksgiving Day, he communicated to all of the clan that he was in fact a licensed pastor turned drag queen who turned tricks for money in Jacksonville, Tallahassee, and Atlanta for many years, mostly to fund his drug addiction. I was shocked, to say the least, because I had made assumptions about that gentleman based on his faith and knowledge of God. And I wondered what could have been going on in the heart and mind of a man, for him to climb down from a pulpit delivering the word of God, and end up sucking penises in a parking lot in a dress for crack rocks? And before I knew it, there I was judging him.

I sat on Renee's couch quiet, but inside, I was puffed up like a proud peacock. It left me for a few moments that I was a transgender woman of color, who also had done some unspeakable things for money, but not because I had an addiction to drugs. And that it was the same grace and mercy of God extended to us both that was the sole reason that I was educated, drug- and disease-free compared to others like me. I prayed right there that the Holy Spirit would subdue the vile serpent of pride.

I have learned personally that it is the grace of God that often protects us from ourselves. I also learned that day that he was functionally illiterate, reading only to a second-grade level. I was flabbergasted! And then it happened.

It was common knowledge in the group that I had been dealing, or many would say not dealing, with what is known as "church hurt." This term, coined by Pastor Emmett Price, refers to the pain inflicted by religious institutions that invariably distances recipients of abuse from their faith-based communities and God.

"What they did to you at New Birth, Jasmine, was a disgrace and certainly ungodly. And I know you have toiled over this situation for a while, but girl, I'm gonna share something with you. They tout a slogan that says that New Birth is the perfect place for imperfect people. And they encourage members every Sunday to join various ministries so your God-given talents can be used to help others. Right?" he said.

I nodded, as tears welled in the corners of my eyes.

"No matter what their church slogan said, or the open invitation for members to not sit on the talent that God gave them, but to use it for His glory," he continued, "when challenged with a transgender church member, they simply didn't possess the agape love they believed themselves to have. And baby girl, no one can give what they do not have. Honestly, you and I both know that you shoulder the brunt of the blame also, Jasmine."

I consciously chose to ignore his last statement and shifted my eyes away. What I did internalize was powerful. It was like the proverbial mic dropped. I learned that day that it was unfair to myself and others to expect something from someone that they simply did not have. Applying that concept in my life as it related to my transition made it easier to let go of friends and family who didn't have it in themselves to accept me, for whatever unknown reason. That burden, if it accumulates to one, ought to be theirs to carry, not mine. The most challenged individuals, I have found, offer the most profound and grounding advice if given the opportunity. That short conversation allowed me to understand the aunt who raised me a little bit better.

A few Sundays after Thanksgiving, my new friend, who bestowed so much wisdom and kindness to me, sadly relapsed. I never heard from him again.

My Aunt Mary was an amazing individual who gave what she had generously. Whether she was right or wrong, she said and did what she thought was honorable and in the best interest of her children. And for these and other reasons, she became the second superwoman that entered my life. Her language of love for me and others was translated through the selfless act of provision. Providing a roof over our head, food in our belly, clothes on our backs and for myself especially the opportunity to get a formal education in a safe, more academically competitive environment.

Mary wasn't homo- or transphobic, per se; she saw sexuality and gender identity through the same narrow lens that influenced her own sexuality as a young, beautiful woman of color growing up in the segregated south. She had a guarded, repressed concept of sex and ultimately all forms of human sexuality.

The first example: When I was ten years old and my sister Tina was six-and-a-half, Aunt Mary sat us both down to give us the much-needed "talk" about the birds and the bees, and the conversation went a little like this...

"Josh and Tina," (one of our aunt's hilarious and endearing character flaws was that she could never bring herself to pronounce anyone's name, or words for that matter, consistently and correctly... pay close attention, my name was Jof) "sit down here at the kitchen table. Your Aunt Mary wants to talk to you about being a freak and sex. Now listen to me very carefully, because I'm not gonna repeat myself about this here," she said as she stood over us with her right hand on her hip and the left resting on the kitchen table balled up in a fist. She glared at my sister and me, leaned in a little closer, and with both hands she grazed over her breasts, crouch and backside in a circular motion, and said without flinching, "All this here is yo' ass. You are to never let anybody come anywhere near yo' ass or your hind parts. Understand? This world is full of freaks and sissies who want to do filthy things to little boys and girls. Okay? You two got that? That's the first thing. The second thing is that older men will give you worms in your guts if you let them play in yo' ass and finish their business. I don't know a single soul who would want worms in their ass, if they could help it, do you? And the last thing I'm gonna say, is the same thing I tell all the churn'n I raise. Don't bring yo' ass back home prignant" (she meant pregnant) "with a belly full, because your Aunt Mary ain't gonna nursemaid no gotdamn babies. Whosoever come home prignant better take their ass back out in the streets where they been laying the f**k up and find a daddy for the bastard growing in their belly, 'cause I'm not taking care of anyone else's responsibility. I'm too damn sick and tired. Got any questions? And if you do, don't ask me a gotdamn thing. Just do as I say and you won't get into any trouble," she concluded.

That whole little speech was a disturbing mouthful. My little sister giggled her head off, but I sat there like a deer caught in the headlights of bad sex education.

Mary had a son named Rome. He was approximately ten years older than me; when I arrived, I was almost eight, and he was around 18. Like his mother, Rome had light brown skin and that "good hair" that black folks are always bragging about. He was built like a defensive tackle, smart as a whip and "didn't take any tea for the fever." Rome was a diehard basketball and football fan with a strong resolute personality he undoubtedly got from his mother.

Aunt Mary simply adored the son she had cared for since he was three days old, and he adored her right back. They had an amazing, fascinating relationship. Rome would fuss at his mother about taking better care of her fragile health, and she would find more and more interesting ways to ignore him. It was their thing. It was his most expressed language of love for his mother. Aunt Mary communicated her love and devotion through food especially prepared for him. I remember his favorite foods while I grew up were dagwood sandwiches and fried chicken breasts.

At first, our relationship was good. He and I were the only males in a house that was full of female energy. In my mind, Rome began to see me as a little brother figure and took me around and showed me things the way a big brother will., One Saturday within weeks of my arrival, he told me to grab my jacket and come with him. He took me shopping at a small men's and boy's clothing store in the neighboring city of Allentown. I'll never forget the jacket he allowed me to choose for myself. "Pick out anything you want, Jof," he said.

I began to rifle through the racks of jackets and coats, instinctively honing in on price tags. I was looking for the cheapest one.

"I said, pick out any jacket or coat you want. Don't worry about the prices," he said after catching me. Hearing that, I quickly made a beeline for the jacket that had captured my attention since we'd first walked into the store. It was burgundy, with all sorts of zippers all over it in the style of the early '80s. It had detachable sleeves and a detachable hood, so I could turn it into a windbreaker or a vest depending on how I wanted to rock it. I loved it and was thrilled that he thought enough about me to give me such a cool gift like that.

Unfortunately, our relationship quickly soured. Like I mentioned earlier: mannerisms and behavior. Over time it became clear that I was a rather effeminate little boy. Although I tried very hard to try to "act like a boy" (whatever that meant), I was comfortable playing jacks, jumping double dutch, and doing street cheers with my sisters Tina and Katherine. (Katherine was actually Aunt Mary's great-niece that she was raising like Tina and me; she was five years older than I was, but we became inseparable for a time.)

Katherine allowed and encouraged me to be me. Tina and I both adopted her as our big sister. Katherine loved music, so we would prance around the house, switching and spinning. Every so often, when the adults weren't looking, I would take the chance to try to be the real me, if only for a few moments a day. Katherine and I used to do a vulgar street cheer that she picked up in Brooklyn before she moved to Bethlehem. We would start off with rhythmic clapping and footwork to the cheer, which was called, "Spell Your Mighty Man." Katherine would start off, "Hey Jof, spell your mighty man, spell your mighty man right now."

"OK! I'll be his ice cream, and he'll be the freak. And if he don't like it. Don't tease. Suck these. Stick it in. Stick it out. With his mighty man jam'. S for superman, he's superfly. My Jordache jeans pulled down to my thighs. I pump my nigga and he pumped me right back. With the M-I-GHTY, M-I-GHTY, M-I-GHTY. Hunch back, jump back, bull's eye," I cheered. I know! I was a kid, ecstatic just to be included with the girls.

My cheering was often out of sync and off beat because I stuttered, but I got my "Mighty Man" in nonetheless. The more Rome saw of that side of me, the angrier and more disgusted he became. I mean, I wasn't crazy enough to let him hear me doing the mighty man cheer, but he saw other things. Before long, he had almost zero contact with me and, when he did, would speak about me in brutal terms. "Faggot ass," "sissy," "punk ass"… or any number of pejorative iterations of the same homophobic sentiment. Those were the only words I heard from him in reference to me throughout my childhood and teenage years, either to my face, but mostly to others within earshot of me. Those memories were psychologically and emotionally crippling. Those encounters, and not just with my cousin, shaped how I saw myself as a person, as an individual trying to navigate the already complicated throes of adolescence and my relationship with the only true God.

My homosexual thoughts and desires kept me up late at night as a kid wrestling with his faith. A strong Christian faith first introduced to me as a toddler by my great grandmother Ford, but one that has proven to be tried and true throughout the course of my life. *Why do I feel this way, Lord, and how come you won't take it away?*, I asked Him in prayer when I was no more than ten years old. *I wish I was a girl so my feelings would be normal. Not even a pretty one, if that would be too much trouble, but just a girl*, I asked God like I had hundreds of nights before. And on that matter, I heard nothing. Had I been infected?

Before I left Philadelphia, a series of incidents happened that possibly changed the trajectory of my development, and which I'll never forget. I was young, because my grandmother Rosalee was still alive, and my mother was taking care of Tina and me. I remember Grandma coming over to visit our two-bedroom apartment on the first floor and taking me in her arms and hugging me.

My Uncle Sunny had hit a rough patch and was living with us, sleeping in my bedroom, which faced the side street. He took the bottom bunk bed, and I slept on a cot on the other side of the room. One night long after my bedtime, the glare of the streetlight was shining into the bedroom, when I heard a knock at the window.

Uncle Sunny got up very quietly and opened the window, and a man crawled through it into my room! I could only see his shadow and his silhouette. He was dark-skinned, with an Afro, and he may have had a beard. Uncle Sunny was very light-skinned, so I could still see his image in the darkness more clearly.

The two of them went over to the bunk beds and sat together on the bottom bunk. They began kissing and getting undressed. Even as a four-year-old child, I knew this was not normal. I could feel that this was not how people were supposed to act. But in my innocence, I probably felt that the mystery man sneaking into my room at night was a greater offense than anything he was doing with my uncle.

They continued kissing and petting, whispering to each other to be quiet. I remember it all very vividly – the sounds of their kisses, and of them performing oral sex on each other. I also remember my uncle catching me watching them. The whole time he had thought I was asleep. "Jof, turn your head," he said. He didn't want me to see what they were doing; he wanted me to face the window.

At first, I obeyed. But I could still hear them smackin', lickin', kissin' and carrying on, so I slowly turned my head back around. Hey, I was a child, and children are notoriously nosy as hell and I didn't want to miss a lick or a stick. I pulled the covers over my head just far enough that I could peek, and I watched them in the moonlight. I couldn't clearly see any genitalia for any length of time. I mostly saw their shadows colliding rhythmically together, moving and shifting in harmony with their sounds. And at some point, I must have dozed off, because when I woke up in the morning, Uncle Sunny was asleep on the bottom bunk bed, and the mysterious man was gone.

The first thing I did was go into my mother's room. I spilled my guts. I told her everything, a real blow-by-blow account, from a child's perspective, meaning I was extra and animated. A man had come through the window and he had gotten into bed with Uncle Sunny and they had been kissing and carrying on. I gyrated my bony hips in demonstration, while I squawked and squealed. The more I told her, the more agitated she became. She was in a hysterical rage by the time I was done. Uncle Sunny was still in the apartment, and she ran out of her bedroom and physically attacked him. I remember being shocked by the violence of the fight. She punched him over and over, calling him all kinds of faggot and demanding that he pack up and get out.

It's important for me to communicate that my mother was not surprised to learn that her brother had been with another man. I'm positive that she knew, an assertion I'd pieced together from later conversations with her. What had upset her was that he had done this in front of me; that he had allowed a stranger into her home, into her child's bedroom. That was absolute boundary crossing.

Section 2 (The Serpent and the Child)

My first real sexual relationship with a man began when I was twelve. Kenneth was the uncle of Katherine and Patricia, and a relative to my Aunt Mary through marriage. He was probably in his late forties when it all happened.

My aunt Mary's sister Lucille passed away. I believe she lived in Brooklyn, and as usual in black culture, everyone from New York came down to Mary's house in Bethlehem for the funeral. Most of her eleven children, and some of their children, were all huddled up at the house in preparation for, during, and for several days after the funeral. It was a terribly sad occasion, but it was how I met my new Aunt Debra and her sister, Aunt Lucille, two of her daughters.

The thing about Uncle Kenneth was that the whole family knew that he had pedophilic tendencies. If they didn't know anything specific for sure, they'd certainly heard plenty of rumors. He had been in and out of jail for various crimes, and his sexual proclivities were an unspoken whisper, a kind of rumor going through that side of the family. But he *was* family, so whenever he was out, he was around, and welcome.

Kenneth was grooming me for years before the incident, the night when we got together for the first time. When I was a young boy, he would do things like rub up against me when I was at the kitchen sink washing dishes, grazing his partly aroused crotch against my behind as he walked past me. No matter how much distance there was between us in the kitchen, he would always find ways for our bodies to touch.

He wasn't reckless; like most predators, he was careful and calculating. He wasn't trying to make his move when I was extremely young, he was just getting me used to being touched and caressed by him. And at the same time, I believe he was grooming me emotionally. For years, he would whisper compliments in my ear, and when my cousin would call me names like faggot, Kenneth would take me aside and say things such as, "Don't listen to what Rome says. That's just how he is. Keep being you, Jof. People are gonna talk shit no matter who you are or what you are. You're smart, talented and cute. But mostly cute." I would smile. "Oh! You like when I call you cute don't you. You see. Now I know how to make you smile."

I don't know. It just felt good to be referred to as smart, talented and cute sometimes. I honestly enjoyed the private attention he lavished on me during the time he lived with us or visited. So much so, I began to flirt back with Kenneth, more and more brazenly. I had become comfortable.

By the time I was twelve years old, I was giving him erections on the regular. At that age, he was already grabbing my hand and placing it on his hard penis any time we were alone. They were stolen moments we would wait sometimes all day to experience. In between the physical contact was a lot of lip licking, obscene body language and mouth reading. But for some reason, the funeral was the first time he saw a real opportunity to come for me…more of me.

I'll never forget the night that we first got together. It was winter, and we lived in an old house that creaked. The stairs creaked. The roof creaked. The windows rattled. We had throw rugs, but we didn't have wall-to-wall carpeting, and the wooden floors would creak. So as a kid sneaking around that house in the middle of the night, I learned how to walk down the hallway without waking up Aunt Mary, and how to descend the stairs for a midnight snack by placing my feet in just the right spots, and slowly hopscotch over a creaky floorboard when we were sneaking in late at night. I knew every inch of the dark hallways of that big old house, and could move through it in virtual silence.

Kenneth was laying downstairs. He was the only person down there, and the whole first floor of the house was dark except for the kerosene space heater in the television room. I saw the light from the heater from the top of the landing. I knew that he was downstairs by himself because we had been down there earlier, watching a movie, and he had given another relative his bedroom to sleep in, since they had come all the way from New York. So I crept downstairs and he turned the TV on again.

I went directly into the kitchen to get a glass of water, then lingered around, engaging in small talk with him. He saw exactly what I was doing. I sat down on the floor, and he laid down on a pallet he had made for himself a few inches away from the kerosene heater, and we talked for a few minutes about literally nothing before he gradually maneuvered his body perpendicular to mine. Before I knew it, he had turned off the space heater, turned off the TV and we were alone in the dark. He unzipped his pants and pulled out his penis. Even in the pitch dark, I could tell that he was extremely endowed. But then again, I was a twelve-year-old little boy, so what did I know.

He took one hand and guided my head down to his penis, holding my neck. I didn't feel forced, but I certainly felt obligated to do what we both had been insinuating for such a long time. I performed oral sex on this middle-aged man. Kenneth was in his late forties, so to me he was an old man. Still, there was something unbelievably thrilling and forbidden about that encounter.

I was downstairs in the dark for a while with him before I heard the floor creaking in the front bedroom where at Aunt Mary slept. I knew she would be coming. I jumped up and turned on the lights, and less than a minute later, my aunt came downstairs. There she stood in the middle of the room, in her quilted pink house coat and slippers. I picked up my glass of water off the side table as if I was just down there for a drink, but Mary Johnson wasn't stupid. Right away, because of what people knew about Uncle Kenneth, she began interrogating me. "Who's down here? Why are you down here by yourself?"

"I was just getting some water, Aunt Mary."

"Gettin' some water, huh? Get your thirsty ass back upstairs, boy! You should not be downstairs by yourself in the f**king dark with Kenneth." She looked around the room, surveying to see what was going on. She paid particular attention to what positions we were in when she walked into the room, what our clothes were doing, and how I just couldn't knock the dumb facial expression off my face. When all of that registered, she said with a pointed finger, "Josh, take your ass back upstairs now."

"Nothing was going on, Mary," Kenneth said. "I was just watching some television when Jof came downstairs, I guess for something to drink. And now I'm being accused of something I didn't do," he continued.

"Kenneth, I'm not accusing, I'm just saying. A child ain't got no business downstairs in the TV room in the dark with a grown ass man, in the middle of the night, while the rest of the house is sleep. Ever! Nothing good is going on in that kind of situation. Nothing! And if I ever find out that you assed around with any of my kids, I'm gonna put you underneath the jailhouse," Aunt Mary said.

"I know you would. Good night, Aunt Mary," Kenneth said.

"Uh-huh," she replied.

In hindsight, it's kind of astonishing – you almost have to laugh. People knew about Kenneth. He wasn't hiding his sexuality, and it was never in question. People laughed and joked about how much of a freak he was, but my aunt still allowed him to live in the house with her...and us. Two small children, growing up in a house with a man everyone knew was a pedophile, or at least had a demonstrated propensity to be a sexual predator. Why? I'll tell you;

because Kenneth was a gregarious individual who was reliable if called upon, and who had the ability to be disarmingly charming if needed. Most predators like him possess some of the same traits.

Society as a whole, but especially African Americans, must strive to do better. We have a history of collectively harboring these kinds of sick, toxic secrets as a culture, foolishly believing that silence will in some way nullify the abuse, cleanse or absolve the perpetrator of all "unrighteousness," and spare the victim perpetual shame. Fortunately, life is not that simple. The life that God gave us is designed to challenge us in the most unconventional and uncomfortable ways imaginable. The notion of health and wellness, mind, body and spirit, requires us to do the work. The kind of work, and the amount of work isn't the same for everyone. I myself hadn't done the work for a very long time; thus, the writing of this book. And so the story continues.

Well, it was that funeral that sparked it, and from that night on, he and I would steal moments together. This went on for years, all throughout my adolescence.

As I say, he was grooming me for exactly this purpose, and in retrospect it's both obvious and shocking, but the reason it worked was that there's a very simple and elemental draw. Children need to be validated and empowered, and when an adult takes them seriously – asks them what they think and really listens to the answer, and compliments them not just on their appearance but on their thinking and behavior – that's an incredibly intoxicating feeling. Beyond that, there's something truly powerful about being sexually attractive to another person. Even as a child on the cusp of adolescence, the realization that you possess the ability to cause another individual to have a physical reaction, to make their penis rise for you is stunning. At twelve years old, I didn't know much about sex, I was likely still operating on a mix of schoolyard myths and my own imagination, but to be able to do that…and when that was combined with the idea that he'd been pursuing me in such a sneaky, teasing way for so long, dropping little hints and making little jokes, I felt empowered. I didn't feel like a weak sissy. I didn't feel abused; I felt like I was the one making the decisions and calling the shots, at least in that secret aspect of my life.

Remember, also, the appeal of doing something taboo. Every one of us has done something we were explicitly told not to do. Every one of us has done something we may not have been told not to do, but knew we weren't supposed to do. It makes your heart pump and your blood race in your veins. The air feels electrically charged. You're more alive in that moment than ever before, at least that's how it feels. And the opportunity may never come again.

That was why I did it. I wanted to see what would happen. I wanted to see how far it would go. And on some level I *did* know what I was doing; I understood the power of my position. Even as a much younger boy, at six years old in a basement playing house and manipulating other boys to gain their approval, I already had some inkling of the power of being submissive. As an adolescent, I was that much more aware of it. And as an adult, I understood that power completely.

Unless you've been in that position yourself, you can't understand. If you've always been dominant, you can't recognize the power of submission. When people are submissive — when they're performing fellatio, for example — outsiders think they're the vulnerable ones. But looked at another way, that's a very powerful position to be in. Because you are the provider of pleasure. And you can give it, or take it away.

From the age of six, when I was first molested by an adult man, all through my adolescence, I understood sex as something hidden and secret. It wasn't just the adult-and-child part, it was also the male-on-male aspect. The world showed me again and again that it thought that was disgusting, so I was surrounded with negative tropes about emotions that I felt, and attractions that I experienced. There was nothing affirming about what I did or how I thought or felt when it came to sex. That's a crucial difference that straight/cis people may not truly understand, because they never experience it. Even if you're not looking for it, even if you're not paying attention, you are shown images and messages about positive relationships between men and women all the time. You see courting, conversation, romance, and everything else, and more often than not it's depicted positively and – crucially – something to want and to strive for.

On the other hand, when gayness was discussed at all, in mainstream media and particularly within the black community, everything was negative. It was nothing to be proud of, nothing to flaunt, nothing to really desire. If you were "that way," and if you couldn't pray it away, you were just supposed to relegate it to some faraway, inaccessible part of your mind. So that was how I saw sexuality. It was a dark, forbidden part of me that no one could be told about.

Eventually, when I began escorting – having sex with men for money – the secrecy took on an even darker edge. Charlie Sheen famously said of prostitutes that he didn't pay them for the sex; he paid them to leave afterward. Don't believe that bullshit about "the girlfriend experience"; most relationships between sex workers and clients are exactly that transactional. I, the client, don't want to have a conversation with you, you're not worthy of a truly meaningful interaction. I want this physical pleasure right now, and afterward, I'm going to pretend (to myself and the world) that things never happened between

us at all. As a child I began to inter-
nalize that mindset, to the point that by
the time I was working with clients, I had
little to no respect for them. I was good
at what I did, but I saw them — and treat-
ed them — like walking, talking wallets.
And they saw me for what I was: a piece
of tail, a good-looking, well-built young
black boy who would do what they wanted.
Many of them were married; others were in
serious relationships. They didn't take me
seriously. I was dessert. And I knew it.
When I began to transition, it became even
more secretive. It was almost a dance.
They didn't want any information about me
to get out, so they were paying me for two
things: to be good at what I was doing sex-
ually, and to be quiet about it beforehand
and afterward.

I never analyzed my profession in any
depth at the time. I was a teenager like
any other; I didn't analyze much of any-
thing in any depth. But I convinced myself
that I was running a business. And I set
rules for myself about dos and don'ts — who
I was willing to see as a client and who I
was not, and what I was willing to toler-
ate and what I was not — and at the time
I told myself it was because I was a hard,

intelligent businessperson merely taking advantage of opportunities thrusted into my lap, but on some level I knew that I was also compartmentalizing my trauma in order to make it okay for me to do what I was doing, mentally and emotionally.

By the time I was thirteen or fourteen, I was seeing men for sex, often in Allentown, the nearest big city to Bethlehem. I won't claim I had a flourishing business going, but I certainly made more money than kids with paper routes or jobs at Baskin-Robbins or whatever. I was seeing the same type of men I would see years later as a trans person. I was a slim, pretty young man, hairless in the face and well-endowed for my age, and men who were on the downlow, bisexual or gay made my client list.

I may not have actually known much, but I was able to figure things out. I pieced together very quickly where to go to meet men. It may sound a little crazy, but young adolescent black boys are always popular with older men- especially white men. They'll call you a nigga and suck your d**k, practically in the same breath. As a matter of fact, it has been my experience and contention that white men and white women will both secretly descend from the comfort and security of the suburbs, and make their way down into the inner city or the projects for two things: drugs and a good piece of black d**k. I've seen folks cough up their last dollar for either or both. And honey, they met up with the right one. I was much obliged to take any available coins off their hands.

I would find clients in the back booths of the adult bookstore, outside and inside of public bathrooms. Fairs were huge moneymakers, and men fishing at Monocacy Creek were all too anxious to take a very expensive thirty-minute lunch break. Even in a small town like Bethlehem, Pennsylvania, you'd find married men cruising public bathrooms in the Lehigh Valley Mall. I could walk in and see men waiting in the stalls - or I could go in and wait in a stall myself. A man would leave his wife outside with the shopping bags, come into the men's room, get some quick head, and go right back to walking around the mall with his family! I know this behavior may come off a little grimy, but things like that happened and still happen in every mall across this country. I've seen it more times than I could possibly recall. I grew up watching it happen.

Sometimes, these men would give me their phone numbers, and I might give them a call. I would give them a free show, and then say, "If you want more of that, you're going to have to pay me." My teenage flesh was just like any other drug: once they had a taste, they were willing to pay for more.

Let me elaborate on the topic of the adult bookstore where I would meet men. I would walk past the racks of videotapes and DVDs, the dildos and other sex toys hanging on the walls, and the "sexy" lingerie on racks, straight to the back where the booths were. Men would enter the booths to watch short videos, paying more or less by the minute. They would give you a look and leave the door open just a crack if they wanted you to come into the booth with them. In certain places, the booths had what were called "glory holes" — a literal hole in the wall between stalls. A man would put his penis through the hole, and someone on the other side would stroke or suck it in total anonymity. As a teenager, I would be there at eleven, midnight, even one or two in the morning, turning tricks in the back of the store. And it was not a slow trickle of horny dudes. These men were shoulder to shoulder.

This level of freakitude is common knowledge in gay and bi culture. This was history, and again it happened in every city in America, and even many of the kind of sleepy small towns where you would never believe such a thing could go on. Even in Bethlehem, which was like a middle American town even though Pennsylvania very nearly touches the east coast of the US, a surprising number of men were pursuing these kind of sexual outlets. I saw my English teacher at one of the adult bookstores in town! He and I became close for a while. I liked him as a teacher, and I was a good student, but after that night, we had a lot more contact. He paid me $150 every time he saw me, and trust me, that was a significant amount of money for a 17-year-old in 1989, especially when you're earning it for just a half hour's work — for something you'd be doing anyway, as a young, sexually overdriven male with hormones raging and a penis that never seems to go down. It was like having a hungry-hungry hippo attached to your crotch.

I attended Liberty High School in Bethlehem, graduating in 1990. I had a great group of friends, many of whom were white, and I'm glad they were, because I found them to be a lot more understanding than even members of my own family. Had I gone to an inner city high school in Philadelphia, for example, I would have undoubtedly suffered a lot of bullying — the treatment I got from my aunt Mary's son, only much worse — and I didn't get that at Liberty. I was rather popular and well-liked. I was one of the theater kids (surprise!), and was voted Best Dressed and Most Talented in the yearbook. To this day, I still talk to many of my beloved high school friends on Facebook.

That said, none of them knew that I was a male prostitute. To them, I was just a popular and well-dressed kid; they had no idea that the majority of my clothing budget came from the sex work. After all, I worked consistently since the age of fifteen, first in retail, at a high-end men's boutique, and in health care as a resident advisor for mentally challenged women, men and children at seventeen. But most of my "real" money came from my clients who would pay me for my services. In hindsight, I probably have shared way too much, but a promise is a promise.

Section 3 (Dispensable Me)

Not long before my eighteenth birthday, I moved in with a trick. I was getting a lot of pushback from my aunt at the time — I was growing into myself, becoming more confident in my identity, and she wouldn't allow me to do certain things. Despite the fact that there were openly gay members of our family, like my uncle Sunny and my uncle Kenneth, she was very much against some of the things she saw me doing and becoming, and I wanted more freedom, so I ran away. I called a man I knew who owned a string of flower shops; he was over 60, and very wealthy. He pulled up to get me in an expensive car. I ran out the door, hopped in, and we zoomed away like I had escaped prison.

He lived in a neighboring town in a very nice house. He had a butler and a cook who came in every day. I had been to my friends' middle-class homes and other places, so I wasn't gawking at the luxury like I was on *The Fresh Prince of Bel-Air* or anything, but it was still far from anything I had ever experienced before.

I learned very quickly, though, that I was just as disposable living with him as I'd been when we were hooking up as worker and trick. The age difference was a real problem, as I was simply not attracted to him sexually. I wanted what he had, not him. He had a nice home, to which I had gained access, but I didn't want his sex, I wanted his money and to live in comfort: to be a house pet, more or less.

We developed a strange relationship, somewhere between stepfather-stepson and sugar daddy-sugar baby. He took me in, set me up in a room in his house, and gave me a ride to school every morning in that fancy car. Even better, he would give me $50 every day for lunch. So I would buy lunch for all my friends, and after school we would go to an old-fashioned lunch counter across the street, the kind with chrome bar stools and a soda fountain and everything, straight out of the '50s. We'd all go there and get burgers.

But the fact that the old man and I were not having sex became a subject of greater and greater tension between us, because I just couldn't get it up for him. I was his

trophy, but he got tired of our relation-
ship eventually — something I should have
seen coming, but didn't.

He worked a lot, and left me alone in
the house, which was a pleasant surprise.
Even though I wasn't a thief, I was shocked
that he trusted me with all of his valu-
ables. Unbeknownst to me, though, he had
cameras everywhere in the house, and I was
being recorded. One day, I brought a young
guy my own age home, and we had a real-
ly nice afternoon that culminated with us
having sex on the kitchen floor. After he
left, I showered up and the following day,
after I got home from school, the old man
confronted me. "Come into the TV room," he
said, and when we were in there, he asked,
"Who was here?"

I lied and said, "No one."

He said, "Oh, I know someone was here."

I continued lying, trying to play it
off. "It was just a friend from school, we
were studying."

He looked disappointed. He pressed play
and showed me the video. There I was in
the kitchen. The other young man walked
into the room, we talked, we kissed, we had
sex…I was utterly embarrassed, and hung my
head. He didn't get angry or scream at me,

but our relationship soured after that day. I was still allowed to stay in the house, but I was quickly demoted. He stopped taking me to school; I had to ride the city bus, which took a really long time, and after a week or two, he told me to leave. I arrived at the house one day to find all my bags packed at the door. And as I was gathering my stuff, a little bit shocked but mostly because of the wound to my ego, another black boy around my height, with my same build, came walking in. I had been replaced. It was like a scene out of a movie. I was too stunned to even be embarrassed, but it was crazy. And the whole thing taught me a very important lesson - that people are expendable, period.

My journey has had a lot of twists and turns, as you've probably already figured out. But even I wasn't prepared for the possibility of fatherhood.

When I decided to actually transition, it was an enormous internal struggle. I was living my life, and enjoying it, but there was always a feeling in the back of my mind, in the core of my heart, that I was betraying my faith. I believed in the Lord and wanted to be a good Christian, but there was a pull within me toward what

I truly believed was perversion and sin. It was a daily conflict, and I tried very hard to overcome it, to abandon the dark side of myself and live the way other people lived, the way straight society told me I should.

I actually met a woman, and we began dating. Her name was Diane. She was from Guyana. She was short, dark-skinned and cute, and she spoke with a very thick African accent. We met when I was in drag; she was the roommate of a gay friend I visited often. He was Puerto Rican, living with his mother Dita, who was a huge fag hag. She loved me, and all of her son's other gay and drag queen friends. We would all get together at their house, eat rice and beans and pork chops and Puerto Rican food, and many of us would get dressed there, because we couldn't do it at home. Our parents were "not about that dressing like a girl stuff," if you know what I mean, my aunt Mary very much included. So we would take our drag stuff over to Dita's house and get dolled up there, because she didn't care.

Diane was pretty and friendly, and with my identity struggles I was open to a straight relationship — or some approximation of one. I'd had sex with girls before and been able to perform. The two of us began dating, and eventually, when I was about 20, she got pregnant. Because of that, I tried to put the whole drag aspect of my life away. I had been living a double life in some ways, except that all my true friends and my girlfriend knew both sides of me. In truth, it was a triple life, because my friends knew my drag self and Diane knew me as her boyfriend, but few of them truly understood the struggles going on inside me, between me and God.

I had been moving toward transition, but I put that on hold when Diane got pregnant. She had two children already, a five-year-old girl and a two-year-old boy. So I put everything aside and she and I moved in together and I tried to actually be a "real man" and a father to these children. All my drag friends thought I was out of my mind – I had been transitioning, and then stopped, all because of a girl. They knew her, and liked her; she was part of the group, but still, they knew who I was, too.

I still didn't really like girls per se, but I was trying really hard to be what she wanted and needed. She was genuinely in love with me, and I was drawn in by that love. I didn't want to have sex with her, not really, but I was drawn to her and loved her as a person. So I struggled. I was still seeing men on the side, but I was trying to be there for her and the kids. But then she betrayed me, in the most awful way possible.

During her fifth month of pregnancy, almost her sixth month, while I was working at a straight job during the day, she sneaked away and got an abortion. I was devastated, because there had been no indication from her that this was her plan. I had been so excited about being a father – I had been picking out names, thinking that finally something was going to be mine and I was going to be able to provide the kind of loving, stable home I'd never had...I kept thinking, *Wow, I'm going to be a father*.

I had been reexamining my desire to transition and everything else about my life. I was rethinking everything about who I was. Children will do that to you, even when they haven't arrived yet. You reevaluate who you are in anticipation of them coming into the world. So when she had that late-term abortion, I was frankly devastated. It was almost worse – an additional blow – when I found out it would have been a little boy.

I never saw Diane the same way after that. We stayed together, but the trust between us was gone. I began to do my own thing, going out and seeing men more frequently, and being a little more obvious about it. Still, we tried off and on to maintain the relationship, and there was still some kind of bond there, even if it was fraying. But then she got pregnant again, and she did the same thing.

The second time, I hit her. I regret it to this day, but I was so devastated by her betrayal, I lashed out. And while we still stayed together, even after that, it was the end. I stopped caring about her at all. I no longer loved her; in fact, I hated her. She had killed two of my children, and after that I didn't care who I cheated on her with, I was just staying in that house until I could find a new place to live. Finally, I got an opportunity to move to Philadelphia, and I resumed my transition. I began dressing in drag again, and stepped firmly and once and for all onto the path that's taken me to where I am today.

My first boyfriend as a transitioning person was…well, he was a wreck of a man. He had just come out after fourteen years in prison, so you can imagine. But he liked me, and he was my ticket to Philadelphia, so off we went.

Philadelphia was a revelation. I saw everything there. I was immediately drawn to the Center City area – South Street, and 13th and Filbert, was where the girls were tricking and where all the gay clubs were. I was so enamored of the girls I saw working the corners; I couldn't believe they were making money out in the open that way. I had understood my little world of adult bookstores and public restrooms, but seeing this brazen sex trade opened up a whole new world to me. I was far too frightened to do it myself, but I learned the ropes by going out to the corners at night and talking to the girls. They were fascinating, hilarious, and maybe most surprisingly of all to me, welcoming to a stranger. In the middle of the night I would see five or six girls out there laughing and joking, walking back and forth in traffic, seducing men in their cars…it was an entire world that came alive after dark, and I was sucked in immediately.

I had also begun traveling to New York from time to time, starting when I was eighteen. I would go down by the piers and walk up and down Christopher Street, drawn by the lights and the action but still too much of a timid out-of-town boy to really dive into the city's gay scene, which in the late '80s and early '90s was omnipresent and so fierce it could be almost frightening at times. The kids who populated clubs like the Limelight and the Pyramid had a kind of punk-rock energy that almost dared straight people to say something.

One night I saw something I've never been able to get out of my mind, and it was, honestly, the one thing that truly made me want to transition. I was walking down Christopher Street, and a flashy drop-top sports car pulled up – a Trans Am or a Corvette, a big American sports car with a roaring engine. A handsome, well-built guy with slicked-back hair and jewelry got out, came around and opened the passenger door for the girl with him. She stepped out and it was like a scene out of a movie. It was like they were moving in slow motion, under lights, with the wind blowing her long blond hair and drawing her dress tight across her large breasts.

She was absolutely beautiful. She was so pretty, passersby saw them and slowed down to stare. It was a jaw-dropping moment for me. And as I watched them, I knew that she was transgender, not because of how she looked, but how she acted. She knew she was attractive, and she gave off an over-the-top attitude and a sassiness, and spoke to her man in a voice that was brassy but affectionate.

Looking at her, I felt the thought come unbidden into my mind – *I think that's who I am*. I wanted what she had. The allure, the intrigue, the indefinable sexiness, all of it. The two of them walked into a store and I stood on the sidewalk frozen with fascination, waiting for them to come out so I could get one more glimpse of that magic. Simply coming out of a car and going into a store, the most quotidian of activities, had become an occasion for flirting and switching and sashaying around and eating up every bit of attention that was available, in this woman's world. I was a few feet away, not lurking, but close enough that I could see her face, and I envied what she had, and knew that she represented what I wanted to do and to

become and to be, and I was not going to
stop until I was her.

Guessing Game

I run. I leap. I catapult off
the balls of my feet.

What am I?

I saunter. I turn. I got a
well of energy to burn.

Who am I?

I bend. I pray. I entreat the
sun to always stay.

Where am I?

I squawk. I squeal. I give
birth to new ideals.

Whose am I?

I ponder. I guess. No safe
place for me to rest.

Can you find me?

I dart. I hide. Waiting for
bigotry to subside.

Do you judge me?

I'm tall. I'm short. I
vacillate with self-report.

Can you love me?

Not a boy. Not a girl. I'm
like an alien visiting your
world.

Can you return me?

Jasmine Christine Ford

2/2/2015

Chapter 3: Give Me Body, Fame, and Fortune

I was 21 or 22 and had moved back to Philadelphia from Bethlehem. I had left Bethlehem to escape my broken relationship with Diane. After learning she had aborted two of my children behind my back, I couldn't stand to look at her any longer. So I returned to Philadelphia to put some distance between myself and those painful memories.

My family may not have understood every decision I made, but as the poet, Robert Frost wrote, 'Home is the place where, when you have to go there, they have to take you in,' so I moved in with my great-grandmother, Momma Gearl. Although initially she was not fond of the idea of her great-grandson dressing like a woman, she allowed me the opportunity to find myself. Her love for me was genuine and unconditional. And in her secret time with the Lord, she prayed earnestly for me to receive clarity and peace regarding my decision. But I wouldn't expect anything less from a devout woman of God.

We grew very close during the time we lived together. Grandma would rise early every morning, prepare her customary Lipton tea with a splash of lemon juice, and escape out to her backyard sanctuary, if the weather permitted, to dive into her Bible study. She'd slip into the WORD like an old, comfortable pair of slippers, contoured to fit. And I witnessed firsthand the fruits of her faith through her strength, resilience, wellness, mind, body, and spirit.

She was a ninety-year-old woman with a perky schoolgirl laugh and wit as sharp as a tack. I loved my great-grandmother deeply. I educated her on the little I knew about modern LGBT culture and the gender revolution I found myself on the cusp of. She educated *me* on the reliability of tradition, hard work, and faith. Oh, granny and I got it in.

She was a deep thinker, and not nearly as narrow-minded as her great-grandchild apparently was. It was not uncommon for her to conclude that I was sadly out of touch with my own culture after one of our profound conversations about life. Which honestly offended the hell out of me. How out of touch must I have been, for my ninety-year-old great-grandmother, born in the throes of racial oppression during the turn of the twentieth century, to be hipper than me?

"Jasmine, I can't believe you think that way, and you were born a man who now lives as a woman. Do you realize that how you think and how you live are totally opposite? You are the most consistently inconsistent person I have ever known. And honestly, I don't know whether you suffer from mental illness or profound foolishness. I let you dress that way while living in my house partly because I feel sorry for you," she said once.

I thought to myself at that moment, *If another elder refers to me as foolish, I'm going to have to seriously examine the validity of that assumption.* Come to think of it, maybe I should not have told my grandmother that I thought sex between two men was an act of extreme barbarism. That lesbian sex looked like a slow death by a thousand tongue lashes, or that transgender individuals were the bottom-feeders, the proverbial cockroaches, if you will, of the LGBT community. I didn't realize at the time why I would burst into unprovoked bouts of self-loathing at a moment's notice. All I needed was an audience of one. All I was playing to was an audience of one — myself. By adopting a "me against them" mentality, I would convince people that I was the acceptable exception.

In hindsight, I realize that her wealth of life experiences allowed her to relate to me so well during the most challenging time in my life. She knew that her great-grandchild was lost, hurting, and searching, but also realized that peace would come only when I'd given it all to God.

One afternoon, I was walking down South Street with a cousin. It was a hot summer afternoon, and I was working a tight floral romper, open-toe sandals, a long bone snatched ponytail, and a lightly dusted face courtesy of MAC.

I had resumed the transition I'd abandoned when I was with Diane. Through the word on the street, I was hooked up with a doctor who had a side hustle of providing hormones to trans girls throughout the area. I was taking Premarin pills and Delestrogen injectable. I was in pursuit of softness like nobody's business. And I was cute, considering. You know, when you first start your transition, confidence and lip gloss will carry you a long way.

As my cousin and I sashayed down the block, carrying on like neither of us had any home training, I spotted a white transgender woman from half a block away. This lady wasn't fooling anybody. I mean, girlfriend couldn't pass for female at a thousand paces in the dead of night and buried six feet deep. She had a rugged John Wayne jawline (the kind that a man's man dreams of), so much heavy foundation that it discolored her collar, and a receding hairline. Her face was as hard as Fort Knox was to break into, and her body wasn't much better. It was so square, she looked like a walking geometry problem.

She was wearing a white lab coat, and was obviously a nurse or a doctor. I couldn't be sure from a distance. But she was speaking to two men who were medical professionals, too, because they had the entire ensemble: white lab coats and green scrubs, and she was in all-white scrubs and a white lab coat. Seeing her intrigued me. She was the first transgender woman I had ever seen in what appeared to be a position of authority.

In the short time I had been transitioning, I'd seen transgender individuals often, but always in varying degrees of powerlessness. I needed to know that we could be so much more. I needed to know who this lady was and what she did for a living.

I walked up to this complete stranger and introduced myself with the courage only the young possess. "Hi, my name is Jasmine, and I just recently moved back to South Philly. I like your outfit. What do you do? Are you a doctor? Are you a nurse? Are you someone who cleans up after a doctor or a nurse?" I asked.

Astonishingly, she was open and friendly, and we had a short but very polite conversation. "I'm a charge nurse in the ER here," she said.

We were standing on the sidewalk in front of Thomas Jefferson University Hospital on 10th and Walnut St.

She told me that she had a master's degree in her discipline. She took time to talk to me even though I had interrupted her conversation with her peers. She appeared excited that I took an interest in what she did.

Her name was Barri because her male name had been Barry, so that was her way of changing her name but not changing her name. I told her, "I really want to get into nursing," and I meant it. I had been searching for a path, and medicine seemed like a good fit for my personality. Nursing could also be my way to a future of financial security, I thought.

Barri gave me her phone number – either on a business card, or maybe I wrote it down – and told me to call her, because she thought she could point me in the right direction. We said our goodbyes, and my friend, cousin, and I kept walking, heading into downtown Philadelphia.

A day or so later, I gave her a call. She lived right in Center City, and she immediately said, "Come on over. I'll make some tea, and we'll talk." And I did! I went to her house, and we spent several hours together chit-chatting.

She led a modest life in a second-floor apartment in a chic neighborhood. The condo wasn't lavish or fancy, but it reflected Barri's personality – it was decorated

like the home of a middle-aged profession-
al woman, who was grossly devoid of style.
But her warm spirit filled her abode with
charm.

As we spoke, I learned quickly that
her transition had cost her a great deal,
both financially and emotionally. She con-
fided in me that she had been married for
35 years to the same woman and had been
a father of three adult children. She'd
waited until middle age to reveal that she
was trans and intended to embark on her
transition.

To her family, this news came out of
nowhere, and they didn't take it well. For
a trans person, the decision to reveal
one's true self to others is both terrify-
ing and tremendously relieving. It's like
dropping weight off our shoulders that
some of us have been carrying for years,
if not decades.

But our liberation can feel like a bur-
den to people we love. Barri had been a
married man, not only a father but a grand-
father. And to see the patriarch of the
family in hair and makeup proved to be way
too much — even for white folks.

It was so stressful, in fact, that Bar-
ri's wife had filed for divorce, and the

children he raised and loved turned their backs on him. One of the three adult children was at least cordial to Barri. Still, transitioning had cost Barri her entire family, for all intents and purposes. Her relatively privileged life would never be the same.

I sat on her couch feeling a little sorry for her, even though she was a gainfully employed healthcare professional. The stress in her life due to the judgment, societal rejection, and the recent denial of a promotion to Director of Nursing was expressed in her countenance. On some minute level, Barri was experiencing, in real-time, what it was like to be black in America, even if that fact went unacknowledged by her.

I have never been one to bite my tongue. I told her exactly what I thought and why I thought it. She marveled at my youthful insight concerning the intersection between race and gender – "intersectionality" being a term she claimed she had never heard before. But it was not my intelligence she was exposed to that day; it was good old black common sense.

"Barri, the fact that you are actually shocked that you are being treated the way that you're being treated is hilarious to me," I said.

"I don't think I follow you, Jasmine," she said.

"Girl, you went from being the son that everyone brags about during holiday get-togethers because of his athletic or academic prowess to being the black sheep of the family. That undesirable that no one wants to acknowledge, never mind introducing legislation that would address the systemic issues that prevent you from totally realizing the American dream. An American dream that you formerly had in the bag," I said.

I went deep on her ass in mid-sentence and put some political stank on it, for good measure. I read the look on her face as it finally sunk in. She was convinced that her intelligence and "good-personhood" afforded her the privilege and lifestyle she had become accustomed to.

Still, despite her own challenges, she gave me some genuinely valuable advice. She said to me, "You're so young and beautiful. Life for you can be different from how it's been for me." She had put aside the idea of living as a woman. She did not want to let anyone down in her family for so long because she didn't want to disgrace her devout Catholic parents or shame her siblings. Growing up in the Sixties had not provided her with the opportunity to truly be herself. She felt I had something that she did not – the internal strength to transition as a young person. I had my entire life ahead of me, and a small piece of her envied me.

She also shared some of her knowledge about the nursing field, advising me on steps I needed to take and what to expect. We kept in contact for a little while after that meeting but eventually drifted apart – our lives were on unique paths, after all. But what stuck with me then, and has remained with me all these years later, was her story. Although exposed to life's disruptive challenges due to her transition, there was still a twinkle in her eye when she spoke about her future as a woman.

After we spoke, her professional advice marinated in the back of my mind. Two years later, I found myself in Miami, enrolled in a nursing program at Lindsey Hopkins Technical College.

Barri was the first person who encouraged me – who believed, and impressed upon me, that there was more to life than being a shape or a sway. Which to me at the time sounded like total bullshit. I thought it was just the kind of thing an old, soured queen would preach to her replacement, but it would take another 20 years for me to understand and appreciate the gift that was Barri.

As a young trans person, especially a trans woman of color, I learned quickly the sizable premium placed on beauty and passability. The pressure to "pass" as a woman or "be real" is overwhelming. It determines your status in society, directly correlating to the level of privilege society will grant you. Your experience of the world can be positive or highly negative — to the point where your very life may be at risk.

It's sad, but it's true. When you're transgender and pass as a woman, society will give you a physical and emotional and sometimes a financial pass. When beautiful, one has more resources at their disposal and more opportunities, translating to exposure to more potential romantic relationships.

When you don't pass, your entire experience as a trans person is punitive — financially, socially, psychologically, and potentially physically. It relegates your entire existence to that of a "thing." You're "not a boy, not a girl, you're like an alien visiting this world." And judging from the last several years, we all know how aliens are treated. Don't we? So passability is the standard or metric that most transgender women measure their entire existence against. And it's brutal.

It's analogous to being a mulatto or quadroon, passing for white. The knowledge that who you are genetically brings a negative social standing within the community to which you belong is a hell of a burden. By passing as a member of the privileged majority, on the other hand, one bypasses all of the negative consequences of being a member of the minority group. But one can wind up with a kind of "survivor's guilt," realizing that others aren't getting the same benefits, just because of their physical appearance.

That sense of isolation and bitterness was foundational to my life as a sex worker. I embarked on prostitution for several reasons: first, I found a lifestyle where men validated me with money to be liberating. Second, it helped me avoid some of the pitfalls that the social rejection of individuals who transition presented. Over time, I fostered my own affirming community of friends, family, and admirers. Third, although I didn't understand it for years, I suffered from the same cluster of self-esteem issues inherent within the transgender population. You don't really notice it when you're in it, but it's still there.

When I was fully involved in sex work – when I had my website and was being featured in adult magazines – it was very flattering. It's intoxicating. It is so easy to be enticed by this new world of sex, money, and secrets. Where you were once called a sissy and a faggot by people around you, now you are the "It Girl" within a secret subculture, the lucrative underground world of high-end prostitution. It's an "eyes wide shut" kind of altered reality. You pass through a tiny, secret door, and an entirely new world is revealed to you.

The amount of money sloshing around the global sex trade is enough to make your eyes water, and the notoriety you can achieve at your peak is stunning. When I was being featured in magazines, men would call me from around the world – from

England, Germany, Jamaica, South America, and across the US — because they saw my photo. That was the power and phenomenal reach of internet sex ads. I was found, out of potentially thousands of providers nationally, to be uniquely beautiful. And I was pursued, catered, and coddled like a celebrity.

When your power and privilege are built on physical attractiveness, one becomes desperate to maintain it, and I kept it for over 25 years.

The bodies I saw on the "girls" in New York and Philadelphia were off the chain. And they were revered and admired in the LGBT subculture for their beauty, and sought after by self-professed straight men like mythical unicorns. I felt as though I'd lived my life from the sideline, and I desperately wanted to know whether the grass was indeed greener on the other side. I know it sounds painfully narcissistic, but I wanted to be the object of people's obsession for once in my life.

I found JoAnn in Harlem, New York, who shot the girls up with premium silicone. If there was such a substance, she had it. JoAnn had an apartment on the seventh floor, I believe. She was a golden tan-complected woman in her fifties, who started out as a nurse working for a primary care physician in the city. This particular doctor pumped the girls with silicone as far back as the late Seventies and throughout the Eighties. Although she wasn't a licensed physician herself, he taught her everything she needed to know about the underground business. She followed his technique to the letter and soon perfected her own style of instant body enhancement. JoAnn told me that she took over his very lucrative practice when the doctor she was working for decided to retire. So lucrative was his business that, in the end, he hardly practiced legitimate medicine.

What I really adored about JoAnn and came to admire greatly was that she was a true artist – an artist who was more concerned with her clients' health and well-being than turning a profit. She would often turn t-girls away who wanted additional silicone placed in their cheeks, buttocks, and hips before giving their body enough time to heal from the previous "surg" session. I understand that she still injected silicone, a substance not approved to be injected directly into body cavities. However, in my opinion, JoAnn could have taken full advantage of individuals inundated with self-esteem and body dysmorphic issues. Especially since she had such a monopoly on the underground art form for so many years before others came along. Almost daily, clients of hers flew into the City of New York from around the country.

I will never forget the first time I met JoAnn. She let me in, and I was surprised to see that her living room was organized like a makeshift doctor's office. It was beautifully decorated with a lot of vintage pieces of artwork and furniture. The living room/waiting room was immaculate, and felt lived-in at the same time. She had a small examining table in one corner. I saw vials of a clear, gooey solution that had the consistency of motor oil, that she would suck up into a tuberculin syringe to do subcutaneous injections into the cheeks and chin. She also used a larger needle designed for intermuscular injections into the gluteus maximus (buttocks), hips, and the vastus lateralis muscle (thigh). Bodywork is usually performed with the assistance of injectible lidocaine to numb the area before a series of intermuscular injections of silicone.

JoAnn donned gloves and used alcohol wipes to clean every surface she or I touched. I found that a bit reassuring. The concept of being injected with a literally unknown substance was far removed from anything I had ever experienced back home in Bethlehem. But I was excited, too. My heart was pounding from the minute I arrived.

I was instructed to sit up straight and totally still on the examination table. I remained motionless as JoAnn began her prep work. Like an artist, she would stand back and study my face from every possible angle to see where I would need to be femininely enhanced. She held the syringe delicately, with two fingers gripping the barrel flange and the palm of her dominant hand gently resting against the graduated tube. She was the Picasso of silicone, and her syringe was her brush. I was her muse, and my body her canvas.

"Okay," JoAnn blurted. "You have really nice features already. All you need to do is get rid of that strong chin and beef up those high cheeks of yours," she said as she held a large mirror to my face.

"Well, whatever you think I need to look pretty, I'm willing to do," I said nervously.

She proceeded to make my cheeks fuller, plumped up my thin Caucasian-ish lips, and rounded my square chin with silicone.

"Now, look at your face from all angles. Making your cheeks fuller and riding the nature bone way into the hairline feminized your face while giving you beautifully slanted eyes," she said with a smile.

JoAnn handed the mirror back to me for me to examine her work. Was the process painful? Absolutely. I would be a complete nut and liar to deny such a thing. Not only did the tiny needle hurt while she poked dozens of tiny holes into my cheeks, lips, and chin, but the sound it made was highly disturbing. Because the needle was injecting silicone into my face, which is close to my ears obv, I actually heard the fluid being deposited into my face. It was a whistling, bubbling, or gurgling sound at some point. Even so, when I looked into that magical mirror, I saw a girl budding before my very eyes, one who had the potential to be absolutely beautiful.

I took an alcohol pad she gave me and wiped the tiny droplets of blood trickling from my freshly punctured wounds. I was bloody but beautiful, and that was all that mattered to me. The pain I had endured and the horror stories I'd heard previously, about silicone injections performed by other underground practitioners, were quickly dismissed.

I pulled down my jeans, climbed onto the table, and turned around with my ass pointed at the ceiling. The real work began. For this procedure, JoAnn used a larger-bore needle with a 10cc syringe to accommodate more silicone. She first used a very long thin needle to inject liquid lidocaine all around my buttocks and down my hips. It burned immediately, and after a minute or so, the stinging and burning sensation went away. She injected me with about 150-200 cc's of silicone on my first visit. And that's a "guesstimate."

When she was done, she used super glue to seal the holes that the large needle had created. She then put a cotton ball on each one to protect the site and keep the silicone from oozing out. She'd let her patients hang out, give them some juice to drink while their bodies recovered from the local anesthesia, and 15 to 20 minutes later, they'd be on their way.

In hindsight, knowing what I know now as a nurse myself, this was an insanely dangerous situation to put oneself in. With everything I know now about how silicone can potentially react in the body and my knowledge of human anatomy as it relates to the major vessels, I would never undergo this kind of reckless procedure or advise anyone else to do it. But back then, I was 20 years old with an invisible perception of my life. I would go back to see JoAnn over the next few years, faithfully.

Transgender individuals invariably suffer from body dysmorphic disorder. The ability to instantly impact how one presents to the world at a relatively affordable price makes underground silicone body enhancement almost impossible not to get involved in.

It became very addictive. I saw JoAnn multiple times a year for several years until I finally relocated to Miami Beach, Florida. Even though I was a regular client of the sought-after and well-respected JoAnn from Harlem, I secretly and carefully employed other practitioners' services when she was not available. Luckily for me, and this is how I know God has blessed me tremendously, I have never experienced any major complications from my back-room medical procedures. Horror stories such as the Fix-A-Flat fake silicone debacle in Miami from 2007-2010 never touched me.

(A trans woman thought it would be more profitable to buy material from a hardware store with the same known consistency as silicone. During the trial, the prosecution determined that she purchased a solution made of cement, superglue, mineral oil, and Fix-A-Flat tire mender and injected that glop into unsuspecting clients for several years, hosting what was known in the transgender community as "pumping parties" where the concoction was used. Hence the name. She subsequently caused the death of a cisgender woman who, according to the assistant medical examiner, died of "massive systemic silicone migration." Other victims experienced prolonged acute health challenges that in some cases left them permanently disfigured.)

In my early thirties, when I was living in Miami, I did begin to experience some of the adverse effects of the silicone I had injected over a decade earlier. With the aging process and gravity, I had started to experience drooping of my cheeks and chin.

I had witnessed this unfortunate issue in other girls before.

I was a lot older and wiser, and would not make my condition worse by adding more silicone above and sometimes directly on top of the existing material. This is what I've seen silicone practitioners convince girls to do all the time in hopes of creating a makeshift facelift with the new silicone. This cheap pseudo-medical intervention doesn't do anything but literally compound the problem by further weighing the face down, adding more volume. This is what gives a lot of trans women that signature "pie face."

But I was in an excellent financial position, so I could afford to see a licensed medical doctor who specialized in corrective plastic surgery. Drs. Richard Galitz and Leonard Tachmes of Aventura Plastic Surgery came extremely well recommended. I had a few wealthy Jewish lady friends who did not play when it came to their beauty care. These doctors were the epitome of professionals. They ran a practice that was trans-friendly. But make no mistake, their expertise did not come cheap. The stuff was cheap to put in but cost a grip to get out.

Dr. Galitz began the two-man marathon procedure, extracting as much silicone from my cheeks as possible, replacing it with implants, and doing the same with my chin. He repaired what was known as a "witch's chin," which I had begun to develop. Hours later, Dr. Tachmes extracted loose, gooey silicone entwined with healthy breast tissue out of my chest wall and replaced the space with 1,000 cc breast implants. That was my first major cosmetic surgery, and it cost over $24,000 cash. And that was after the kind doctors loaded me up with a bunch of discounts.

Later on, I also had a tracheal shave in Tampa, Florida, that reduces the structure in the throat, commonly known as the "Adam's apple." No matter how beautiful or shapely a trans woman was, if a guy only had to peep at a neck to determine someone's gender, that was a big problem that had to be rectified. After the swelling went down, my smooth, supple, suckable neck was ready for its close-up, Mr. DeMille. And for a time, because I had issues, I went throat first everywhere I went. I began wearing the short Halle Berry haircut because my tiny neck could carry such an unforgiving style. I found myself laughing gaily for no reason at all but to throw my head back and graze my neck with my hand like an old Hollywood actress. They called it overacting, but I called it pulling a Jasmine. I pulled a Jasmine every time I got around any trans who looked like they had walnuts lodged in the center of their necks. In hindsight, I did many things to intentionally make people feel uncomfortable and self-conscious around me. It was my most cherished defense mechanism.

My riskiest underground medical procedure was actually performed, believe it or not, by an actual physician. This is an oldie but goodie. I never tire of telling this crazy story.

It was 1994, and I was living in Philadelphia with my great-grandmother. I wanted to have an orchiectomy, which was the removal of my testicles. I had heard from others that the procedure would help my body feminize a lot faster. So obviously, I just had to have it done. My goal was to be as soft and as delicate as a daisy, and if that meant chopping my nuts off, well, a girl gotta do what a girl gotta do.

All of the girls in and around Philadelphia used this old white surgeon who apparently lost his medical privilege or license due to fraud or malpractice. I'm not entirely sure about the nature of the scandal. Dr. Spector had to have been in his mid-seventies at least when he was practicing medicine without a license by providing transitioning girls hormones. I saw him biweekly for a two-week supply of Premarin, a form of conjugated estrogen taken orally, and a shot of Delestrogen.

Dr. Spector did exceptionally well financially for an unemployed doctor. Very few medical providers at that time were treating trans-identified individuals seeking gender-affirming care. He was it, and girls traveled far and wide for his service. And they brought cash because disgraced surgeons don't take insurance.

After being on hormones for a few years, I opted to do the orchiectomy with Dr. Spector. I spoke a lot to his houseboy, who instructed me on what to wear to the home that morning, how much cash to bring, and to travel with someone for moral support.

My boyfriend at the time was named Sean. He and I went to the surgeon's house early one Saturday in the middle of summer. Philly was uncharacteristically hot that year. We walked up to a big house that was more than a little run-down on the inside. Not at all like the clean, glamorous Manhattan apartment where I'd gone for my face and bodywork. It wasn't a full-on Rocky Horror Picture Show, but it was definitely a runner-up. And that damn slew-footed, Uncle Fester-looking, emaciated negro houseboy certainly didn't put my mind at ease a single bit. He glided through the house, in and out of rooms like a ghost. I forget what his name was, but he was *creepy*.

Nothing was sterile; the "surgical suite" was Dr. Spector's dining room. He did have a surgical bed and glass jars of cotton balls and surgical equipment that one would need to perform medical procedures.

"Follow me, Mrs. Jasmine," the houseboy/medical assistant said, as he crept up behind my boyfriend and me as we sat in the waiting room.

"You did like the doctor told you, right? You didn't eat anything after midnight, correct?" he asked.

"Yes, that's right. I haven't had anything to eat since last night. I don't want any complications," I said as I followed him across the room into the dining area.

I didn't sign any documentation. I never put my name on anything that would confirm that I was even at his house that morning. I just pulled out $800 in cash and sat on the examination table. I was soon naked, my legs propped up in stirrups as if I was a woman having a gynecological examination.

Dr. Spector entered the dining room from behind a bedsheet that separated one room from another. "How are you feeling today, young lady," he asked.

"I'm okay. Just super nervous," I responded.

I surveyed the room skittishly while he unwrapped what appeared to be several stainless steel instruments and laid them on a side table on top of a sheet of disposable chucks. As I sat there waiting, I wrestled with the thought of calling the whole procedure off. But I didn't. He already had my money, and I didn't know how to ask for it back.

He stepped between my legs. For the first time, I could smell him. His underarms and clothes had a pungent vinegar smell. With a shaking hand, he injected me with a local anesthetic. I want to reiterate that again, for those who are a bit slow on the uptake: local anesthetic. Dr. Spector stuck five or six extremely long needles into my groin to numb the area down to the pelvic bone. I screamed in pain at the top of my lungs. Tears streamed down my face. The needle traveled through my testicular sac, past my groin muscles, and into the nerve bundle to anesthetize me.

"Sean," I screamed. "Sean!"

"I'm here, Jaz," he yelled through the thin walls.

"Breathe, sis. The hard part is almost over," said the lover/houseboy/medical assistant.

"Just one more, sweetheart, and that will be it," Dr. Spector said.

After the shots, I laid back on the examination bed for about a half hour, waiting for the local anesthetic to take effect. Almost immediately, I experienced a warm, almost burning sensation in my groin area and throughout my body. I felt dizzy and light-headed. I could hear my pulse beating loudly in my ear as the walls around me reverberated on beat.

Finally, when I was completely numb from my stomach to my thighs, Dr. Spector emerged from behind the bedsheet made into a curtain. I watched him take a scalpel, cut me open, clamp down my exposed testicles and extract them one by one. Testes are a light grey in color, by the way, once you wipe all of the blood off. He stitched me up back up, and I left without them. All because I needed to be pretty. Being pretty was supposed to restore me in ways Jof could not. And so I waited earnestly on the great restoration that never came.

When it was all said and done, I had four breast implant surgeries, three nose jobs, 17 silicone injection procedures, two silicone removal procedures, two chin reconstructions with implants, an orchiectomy, a trachea shave, total facial feminization, a mini facelift and a partridge in a pear tree. Minus any semblance of restoration of any kind. As a matter of fact, to add context to my statement, after every major surgery, I would leap out of bed, run to my full-length mirror, snatch off my fresh bandages and stand there naked. Waiting.

In retrospect, I thought I was trying to achieve an elusive look, but all along, I was waiting to experience a particular feeling, not a look. I had been waiting for the feeling of self-love and acceptance. I had been waiting for the feeling of being enough, just as I was. And I added and subtracted from my body for over 30 years, trying to find the right combination that would grant me access to love, peace, and happiness. I am sorry to say that such treasures were never found on the other end of a surgeon's scalpel. Not for me, anyway.

Ugly

I'm ugly.

I'm ugly because folks say I am.

And I never once rebuked it, or tossed it away,

like the lie I suppose it once was.

As a matter of fact, I held on to it,

Clutched it tight to my bare breast, and I breathed on it.

It suckled at my tit like a brand-new babe, until it drained me dry. Don't ask me why, but I dressed its nakedness in the raiment of my dignity and self-respect.

Oh, it got good wear out of
me.

It got good wear out of me,
until I frayed a t every
seam and broke.

I'm ugly.

Ugly, like the pink liver
stain in the crease of my big

black lips that showed up one
day last summer and stayed.

Like the most base of Negro
surnames; like Jones or
Johnson, it followed me.

It followed me on whispering
lips and echoed in the
ghostly

gaze of strangers as they
strolled by.

This darkness, that I had
once nursed ever so sweetly,

now hovered over my head like
a halo of hate,

and fell upon me daily, like
a steel mesh shroud.

And me,

Too complacent in my pain to
utter a single sound.

I'm ugly.

I'm ugly because the darkness
howled it into my hearing,
and it stuck.

And sprouted big brazen roots
that wormed down deep and
anchored my soul in soured
soil

that I fertilized with my own
self- pity and doubt.

Oh, a hollow place,

Where nothing g r o w s and
nothing's about.

And this locution has dug
lines in my face and scars
down my back.

This affliction that I own
makes it easy to part my
thighs   wide, to entertain
the slight provocation or a
"how do you do?" from a man.

If only to quiet my queerest
sense of consternation.

I'm sho' nuff ugly.

I'm ugly because even the
provincial preacher man,
pandering his pedantic wares
of grace and salvation, cut
his eyes from mine, as he in
finely pressed tweed bops on
by.

Hiding his hellos under
sweat-stained arms

Like big grand Sunday news,
heard on a musty Monday
morning.

What they say?

"A day late and a dollar
short."

I'm ugly.

I'm ugly because I say I am.

And, I won't rebuked it, or
tossed it away,

Like the lie I suppose it
once was.

As a matter of fact, It
swirled around my mouth like
warm tomato soup, and I drank
every drop.

J. C. Ford

2015

Chapter 4: Fractures

Trauma is defined as "an emotional response, of varying degrees, to a particular or a series of difficult circumstances that causes acute emotional and psychological distress such as a car accident, sexual abuse or a natural disaster."

The long-term effects of trauma can be catastrophic if it is not attended to professionally. And just like many people, I never properly unpacked the series of events I experienced as a child, an adolescent, or even as a young adult that caused me irreversible harm. Being gay alone was a shame I just couldn't shake or barely tolerate. And I, over time, accepted the narrative projected onto me: that I was a sexual deviant, perpetually destined for hard times, and on the road to nowhere fast.

I realize that this may be a startling assertion to convey after revealing the sizeable bounty I've garnered during my outrageous exploits in the sex industry, in the previous chapter. Through that maladaptive behavior, I realized much later in life that I was trying to carve out a semblance of a decent life for myself. A life that everyone I knew said couldn't be obtained with their words, their expressions, and their judgment. Impossible? Absolutely! It was akin to trying to build a house out of straw, in the middle of a perpetual sandstorm, while naked. And over the years, "this locution dug lines in my face, and scars down my back" and that darkness "sprouted big, brazen roots that wormed down-deep and anchored my soul in soured soil."

I named this chapter "Fractures" because as an individual who identifies along the LGBTQ continuum, I have experienced cracks, breaks, or fractures in the non-physical spaces of my humanity that robbed me of my peace "which surpasses all understanding," my spiritual gifts given to me by the Father, the sheer joy and benefit of living a purpose-filled life, and my intimate relationship with my Lord and Savior Jesus

Christ. Through poetry and prose, I will finally and publicly reveal some of the most painful memories from my past that had paralyzed me spiritually for a signif-icant part of my life. I hope to finally seal the many fractures in my soul that have conspired to rob me of life itself. "The ugly," as I've named it, "that I had nursed ever so sweetly" in the very bosom of my soul, took root at six years old.

Section 1 (The Letter)

I'll never forget the look on my moth-er's face. Remember Michael, my childhood friend from Winton Street I introduced to you earlier? At some point, I developed a crush on him. There was obviously no sex-ual element to anything; neither of us had any idea what sex was. I certainly didn't, anyway. All I knew for sure was that I really liked Michael a lot, and I wanted to tell him that. I did not realize that there could be anything wrong with that. In my head, my feelings felt very normal and genuine.

I was in Grandma Ford's living room, drawing him a picture, as children do, and it said, "I love you," because that was what love was about as far as six-year-old me knew. My mother was in the kitchen, but she wasn't really paying attention to what I was doing. I was occupying my time. That's about all she knew. Whenever I asked her how to spell this or that word, she would tell me, but she wasn't leaning over my shoulder to see who I was writing to. She was mostly just happy that I was engaged in something constructive. That's what makes a mother happy.

When I was done, I told her I was writing a love note, or perhaps a love letter; I don't remember my exact words, but I offered to show it to her. She smiled broadly and began cooing, telling me how cute she thought my behavior was. I was fidgeting around. I was so excited. She said, "Oh my Goodness, Jof, you've got a little crush... who's the little girl?"

I said, "It's not a girl, It's Michael."

Her face changed in an instant. I watched it happen. When she thought I had a crush on a little girl, she was warm and gooey. When I told her it was the little boy I ran across the vacant lot to play with every day, her expression warped and contorted. I saw something almost like fear in her eyes. And then she grabbed my arms and shook me. "No, no, no!" she said.

I was only six and had rarely if ever seen my mother as upset as she was at that moment. She was usually more balanced when she dealt with me.

"No!" she said again, her tone cutting like a blade. "You can't like a boy! You can't like a boy! You can't give him this, Jof," she said. Then she elaborated: people won't like you, they will hurt you, this is not good, and on and on.

It terrified me. "I'm sorry, Mommy," I said. "I'm so, so sorry. I won't give it to him, I promise." She was so upset, and I just wanted to take her pain away. I knew I had caused her pain, but I honestly couldn't comprehend why. I heard why. But I didn't understand the gravity of the moment.

Once I told her I wouldn't give Michael the letter, she relaxed a little and let me go. Of course, being a child, I got away as soon as I could and did precisely what I'd told her I wouldn't do. I sneaked across the vacant lot and put the letter into the mail slot at his house. I was so excited to tell Michael how I felt about him, even though my mother had told me not to. Oh, how I wished I had listened.

By the time I slithered back over to Cantrell Street, Mrs. Evans, Michael's mother, was already on the telephone talking to my mother. My mother did a lot of listening, throwing in the occasional, "uh-huh" and "aha!" She never once took her eyes off of me as I stood in front of her, panting and winded. She hung up and simply said, "come on, Jof, we're going over to the Evans."

I had been friends with the Evans boys for quite some time. I remember going on summer outings with the entire family. They saw me as an extended member of their family and showed me kindness as often as they could. Mr. and Mrs. Evans, who sat on their davenport with their son by their side, didn't offer a smile between them that day. The letter severed that relationship permanently.

This was the heart of the conversation.

"Jof, Michael got the letter you put in the mail slot, and it is really concerning. We are trying to raise good strong boys, and the behavior that your child is trying to inject into our family just can't be tolerated, Carla. What's wrong with your son?" Michael's mother said.

Lines of disappointment and disgust were deeply etched into her face. Her furrowed brows were like wide horizontal trenches that seemed to wrap around her entire head. Her whole body frowned at me as I sat next to my mother. My mother felt it too. She quietly reached for my hand, held it, and squeezed as tight as my little hand could stand.

Tears welled in my eyes and ran down my smooth brown face. Shame in its purest form filled every crevice of my body, like dirty rainwater seeping through cracks in old asphalt. Suddenly, I felt like something else, something vile, slithery, and low. I disappeared right before their very eyes, mind, body, and soul. And my childhood innocence buckled under the weight of their grown-up judgment. But the woman who I disobeyed spoke up on behalf of her trembling child — the son she loved and had to protect.

"First of all, Karen, you need to take that chastising tone out of your voice — talking to my son like you're crazy. Jof didn't mean any harm by writing little Michael the letter. That's his innocent way of expressing how much their friendship means to him. I read the letter myself. He just told your funny-looking son how cute he was. That's all. These are children. Little boys and you're talking to them like they're grown-ass men who you caught doing something terribly offensive or even criminal. I told my son not to give the letter because I knew how it was going to be misinterpreted," my mother said.

"Well, if you feel that way, Carla, our kids never have to play together. Because I can't help but see a pattern here, beginning with your brother Sunny," Mrs. Evans said.

Michael sat with his head hung low, and never looked up at me through the entire conversation until then. We both had tears in our eyes.

"Get up, Jof. Let's go. And Oh! You see a pattern, huh? Well, I dare you to tell my dizzy-ass brother that to his face, so he could barrel down Winton Street like a Tasmanian Devil and wouldn't stop until he made it straight to your muthaf**kin' front door. Do not play with me. Don't get knocked the hell out in front of your pretty family. That would be a really messed-up thing to do, and I'm just that messed-up to do it, too, and care not. Everybody on this block knows that Carla Ford is as cuckoo as a cuckoo clock. And I will kick ass every hour, on the hour, when it comes down to my kids."

My mother mumbled all kinds of obscenities under her breath as we walked north on Winton. She had me by my hand, walking as fast as my legs would go, marching as though she was going to war. When we were some distance away, she stopped, swung me around directly in front of her, and yelled, "Never do that again, Jof. Listen to me the next time; damn."

I hung my head and cried out, "I'm sorry, Mommy. I'm sorry."

"You're too young to understand, but people are going to treat you differently if this is who you are, baby," she said in a much softer tone as her eyes became glassy. "And stop hanging your head all the time. You did nothing wrong. Don't worry, you'll meet new friends to play with, and for goodness sakes, stop telling every little boy that you play with that they're cute. Keep that to yourself until you understand what your feelings really mean. Understand?"

"Yes, Mom," I said with a smirk.

"Jesus, Jof, we gotta find you some ugly-ass friends; otherwise, we're going to have to move out of South Philly after-while, with your fresh self. And I ain't got no money to move. My baby boy is about as crazy as his mother," she said with a chuckle.

Michael's parents made good on their promise. We never played with one another again. Even though my mother handled that childhood crisis with the tender loving care only a mother could display, she could not prevent it from becoming one of my very first fractures.

Section 2 (Showerman)

The second fracture came shortly after the first.

One day that same year, my mother, her sister Lisa, and a few of our neighbors were sitting outside on the porch, talking away the afternoon as adults always seem to do when you're a child.

I was told to fetch Aunt Lisa's boyfriend because it was time to eat. He was in her house, so I walked the short distance down the block and went inside. I could hear him upstairs, in the shower. I knocked on the door and said, "It's Jof; I have to use the bathroom."

He told me it was okay, that I could come in. He was in the shower, and I was naturally curious about the sight of a nude adult body. He saw me looking at him and said, "It's okay; we're both boys. It's okay to look. Soon you'll be a grown boy, and you'll have a body like mine," things like that. He was dark-skinned, muscular if my memory serves me correctly, with bushy hair and a thick mustache/and-or beard. I peed, and he finished his shower, stepped out of the tub, and dried himself off, and went into the front bedroom to dress. He called for me to follow him. I was an obedient child, so I went where I was summoned.

He was getting dressed, but when I entered the room, he stopped. "Come over here," he said.

I walked closer to where he was standing. He let the towel that was around his waist fall to the floor. I just stood there looking at him. I knew I shouldn't be there, but I was too afraid to run. I was paralyzed with fear.

"If we do something, do you promise not to tell your Aunt Lisa or your mother?

Because I could get into a lot of trouble, and your aunt won't want to see me anymore."

I never gave an audible answer. The man wasn't waiting for consent from a child, but for the child's struggle-free compliance. He looked at me and asked me to pull my shorts down. I did as I was told. I pulled my shorts and underpants quickly down to my ankles.

I don't remember, honestly, whether he made me do anything to him orally. I only remember the sodomy. And even that's too painful to contemplate.

The whole encounter seemed to play out in slow motion. It was awkward. I had no idea what I was doing or what he was doing. He manipulated my body like a delicate marionette, whispering his approval into my ear as he laid me on my stomach and hovered over my naked body. I remember being very aware of his cologne, the smell of it filling my nose as he loomed over me. This adult man slowly pressed down on me with the total weight of his body.

He was extremely heavy. I could hardly breathe. I remember the feeling of the bedspread pressing into my skin as I lay face down. I remember him putting a glob of Vaseline, or possibly hair pomade, in the crack of my butt and pushing himself against me. I couldn't move.

I struggled and screamed, but he cupped my mouth with his big hand. I remember the sensation of my tissue tearing, the initial feeling of being invaded, and burning pain. With my face toward the bedroom hallway, I prayed for someone to come help me, but no one did.

It didn't take long for him to be finished with me. He made a low grunting sound, his breath became heavier and more forceful, and then he pushed himself off me. I thought I had wet myself when I felt a warm fluid trickle down my skinny little leg as he moved away and the air in the room breezed across my skin. It wasn't pee; it was bright red blood.

I cleaned myself up as best I could. I didn't know what had happened; I had no reference point to process it. At six years old, what child can process the idea of putting a part of your body inside another person's body? Especially *that* part of someone else's body? For pleasure?

Once again, he told me not to say anything, but it was the way he said it that lingers in my memory. He didn't seem panicked or nervous. It was like nothing out of the ordinary had happened. He got his clothes together and washed with a rag and started the strangest conversation. He was not speaking as someone who had just raped a child.

"So, how's school, little guy? I hear you're a bit of a genius. Yeah, I didn't like school much myself," he said calmly.

I never told my mother. I told no one. That night, I tossed my soiled underpants in the trash. My body began its healing process, but my soul sustained wounds that no earthly source could heal.

The Deep

The Serpent sings softly in
my ear.

It sings the sweetest elegy.

Melodic lies of love serenade
my soul,
And inhibition falls as dead
weight beside my feet.

I come undone.

I become like its prized
steed. Subdued. Bridled.

And mounted with the cruelest
irreverence.

Its pulsating pelvis
stimulate me. Intoxicate me.

We gyrate madly in a sadistic
dance of dissonance,

-Master and slave.

I float freely in the frigid
blackness of its eyes,

my soul takes on water.

Fathom by fathom, I fade.
Until,

Gurgling sounds of ecstasy,
is all that remains of me,

As I   sink   into   the
deep.

-J.C. Ford

Bessel A. van der Kolk once wrote, "Traumatized people chronically feel unsafe inside their bodies: The past is alive in the form of gnawing interior discomfort. Their bodies are constantly bombarded by visceral warning signs. To control these processes, they often become experts at ignoring their gut feelings and numbing awareness of what is played out inside. They learn to hide from themselves."

When I was seventeen years old, I discovered gay nightlife. Allentown had nothing on the iconic gay clubs one would expect to find in New York City or Philadelphia, nor did it provide the safety in numbers that gayborhoods such as Boys' Town in Chicago, Christopher Street in Manhattan, or West Hollywood. But we had a sliver of representation in a club called the Stonewall on 10th Street and a much less conspicuous hole in the wall I affectionately called the Shoe Box, on Hanover Avenue.

In Allentown, the Stonewall club was a knockoff of the historic Stonewall club in Manhattan, where patrons had fought back against tyrannical homophobia perpetrated by the NYPD on June 28th, 1969. The doorman at Allentown's Stonewall club often carded, and the patrons were usually a lighter hue than I preferred in the days, if you know what I mean. So, the Shoe Box it was.

I would frequent that club almost every Friday, Saturday, and Sunday, encountering the usual suspects — white, middle-class gay men, whom I would never seriously entertain as possibilities. I loved to dance, and would dance with anyone if it allowed me to steal the dance floor's spotlight. Patrons would ply me with Sprite or Coca-Cola and drool as I slowly gyrated to Prince's song "Darling Nikki" in front of the mirror surrounding the stage. I danced like a freak on two feet, and I allowed them to bask in the glory of my tart, sweaty youth.

At seventeen, I had an avid appreciation for and attraction to a particular subcategory of gay men, known as the "homothug." That hyper-masculine image of black men in saggy jeans, Timberland boots, and a facial expression that screams, "I wish the f**k you would" teased every one of my senses. It is not lost on me that that description is a thoroughly racist and stereotypical trope of black men that I have been on the receiving end of. At seventeen, my small five-foot-seven frame yearned for attention, and attention I got.

He walked in. He was tall, heavy on the black, and beyond beautiful. He seemed over six feet tall, wore a low-cut beard, and had dazzling white teeth that could be seen even in the dimly lit club. He honestly looked like an out-of-town straight guy who had inadvertently stumbled into the wrong bar. But he didn't appear to be drunk or high.

He meandered over to the bar, ordered a drink, and eyed me on the dance floor. I kept thinking to myself how deliciously out of place he appeared. Whatever he was selling, I was buying. And I wanted it super-sized. And then it happened!

The DJ must have shot himself up with an injection of soul because suddenly, out of the speakers blared "Superwoman" by my girl, Mrs. Karyn White. I glanced over at double-dip chocolate, and he motioned for me to dance with him, not on stage but in the bar's corner. The closer I got to him, the more I could see his strong muscular frame through the tan sweater he was wearing. He grabbed me and spun me around so that we were dancing with his crotch pressed firmly against my butt. He was one of those fast-moving freaks.

I noticed right away that, for a brother, he certainly didn't have much rhythm. Although he was off beat, his hips got the job done. And "We gyrated madly in a sadistic dance of dissonance." I was mesmerized. My mind was cloudy, my hands were clammy, my heart was pounding, and I was weak in the knees. I didn't know whether to pop a boner or faint, so I compromised with a breathy question. The first verbal exchange between us of the evening.

"Hi, my nana-name is James, but some people call me Jamie," I said.

"Well, which name do you prefer me to call you?" He asked.

"Jamie," I responded. "James is a little too masculine and less alluring for my taste, but that's a whole other, confusing story. So, how old are you?" I asked.

"I'm 38. Is that too old for you?" He said.

My inner voice screamed, *Hell no, daddy dearest. I'm game, as long as poppa don't preach.*

A half dozen ageist jokes and one-liners from music and movies flooded my brain. I often retreated to movie dialogue when I was nervous. "No, your age doesn't matter to me. Besides, you look fantastic for 38. You must work out incessantly," I said.

"Incess-what?"

"A lot. You must work out a lot. A great deal," I clarified.

"Well, a brutha does, what a brutha can do," he said with a smile.

The music seemed to fade into the background as we conversed. I focused mainly on his full lips that were only a few shades lighter than his smooth cocoa-brown complexion. And when his lips parted wide enough, two perfect rows of bleached white teeth twinkled in his mouth. His beautifully chiseled cheekbones, square jawline, and sculpted body did everything for me. That man was movie magic, cinema-tastic. A casting director's wet dream. Reel by reel, he reeled me in. He peeled me thin. I clung to every word that bounced out of his handsome mouth.

He revealed his name was Marc, spelled with a "c," and he was a truck driver from the west coast who often passed through the area, delivering supplies. It wasn't peculiar how vague Marc was about his last name, the actual name of the city he was from, or what company he drove for. People tend not to overshare with strangers in dark, sweaty bars. So, what he didn't offer, I didn't ask. In hindsight, my misjudgment of character almost proved to be a fatal mistake.

"Um, anyway, can we go somewhere else and get better acquainted," Marc said.

"Well, sweetie, the fates have cast us in the black gay version of *Cinderella* because I, the damsel of your dreams, begrudgingly, have to leave. Curfew! And don't laugh, but my curfew for this evening is midnight…give or take," I said, referencing the clock above the bar. "I really only came out to dance a bit. I didn't think that I would actually meet someone that attracted me tonight. But none the less, *Nous devons donc maintenant nous separer de mon amour*," I said, prying myself from his arms.

"Oh shit! The buttery nigga speaks French now?" he said with a laugh.

"Only enough to get me laid. I mean, that was the whole gist of the French Renaissance, right? Great art meets great sex," I replied, putting on my goose-down jacket.

"I get it. You're smart. You browbeat people with your intelligence to mask your insecurity about being a skinny, gay, black boy with a stutter. The old 'eat before being eaten' syndrome. Classic! It's the hallmark of the most tragic of tragedies. You're not the only one who can disarm people with puffed-up words, with the flick of a sharp tongue," he said.

"Oh wow! R-r-r-really? And which off-brand cereal box did you pull your whack-ass psychology degree out of, Marc? Oh, I get it. You must be one of those trans-formers. You know, the kind that starts off as a really nice guy but turns out to be a catty, sad queen wearing a man suit. Now, I really must go. I don't have a wick-ed stepmother, but I damn sure got an Aunt Mary," I said and flounced out of the side exit.

It was 11:30 PM. I had 30 minutes to walk five miles in the brisk mid-November air. I had just missed the last city bus that left Allentown, heading towards Beth-lehem on the Hanover Avenue route. I had only gotten a couple of blocks away from the Shoe Box when a car pulled up just in front of me. It was Marc.

"Get in, Jamie. I'll give you a ride home. I'm sorry for the things I said. I really like you," Marc said.

I looked down Hanover Avenue, dreading the long walk ahead of me. Something tugged in my gut. Intuition or the Holy Spirit; whatever it was, I ignored it, exhaled, and got into the car. I remember him having an enormous dog in the back seat. Marc said he was a special breed of Doberman that was his faithful companion during his long, lonely road trips. He was being nice again, so I didn't mind when he asked me if we could stop to let the dog relieve himself and stretch his legs. I thought twenty-five minutes was more than enough time to stop for five minutes and get home in time.

We stopped at Woodlawn Memorial Park, a large cemetery on Airport Road. Funny, the cemetery was in the opposite direction from my house. I was now about five miles past the club. The area was pitch black and relatively secluded at nearly midnight in November. A yellow neon sign that read Royal Motel cast a haunting light onto the first few rows of gravestones, only about 20 feet in front of us. Marc and I sat on the little hill, on the grass, in the cold. The dog vanished into the dark cemetery, beyond the reach of the neon sign.

He pulled me closer to him, and we kissed. At first, it felt nice, almost romantic. Then he fumbled with my zipper, trying to unzip my pants. Even then, I was still having a good time. In my head, I thought I could control the momentum of whatever was, or was not, going to happen between us that night. I was wrong. Every time I would remove his hand from trying to unzip my clothes, he would counter with additional force, pressing his weight firmly against me until he was on top. Kissing me frantically. I couldn't catch my breath. At that moment, I realized that not only did I not have control of the situation, but I had in fact relinquished any control the second I got into his vehicle. And I was a little scared.

"Stop. Stop. Stop. I really have to go," I said, as I used every ounce of my strength to push him off me.

"Are you sure? I'm having such a good time," he said.

"We really have to go. I'm super late and going to get in a lot of trouble if we don't leave now."

"Okay. Okay."

His dog was nowhere in sight. He'd descended further into the cemetery earlier and hadn't made a sound since.

"Here, boy!" Marc called. He called again into the cold blackness, "Come here, boy." There was a short interlude of silence. "He's not coming. Please help me find him," he said.

"In a dark cemetery? You want me to help you find a dog in a cemetery in the middle of the night? Hell, no!"

"The sooner we find him, the faster I can get you home. I'm not gonna leave him, and we can't wait for him. I know my dog; something caught his interest out there," he said.

I was hotter than fish grease. "Alright! Come on," I said.

We headed down into the dark cemetery as both of us called for his dog. Woodlawn Memorial Park was a beautiful cemetery. Although I had walked the grounds a few times by day in my youth, the lay of the land at night was beyond frightening. As far as I could see, tombstones of granite, marble, and stone, new and old, jutted up from the cold, stiff earth like bones. Tall trees with wide bulging trunks were scattered throughout the field.

We made it to one of the largest trees in the middle of the cemetery, far from the streetlights that lined Airport Road. "Come, Baron. Come, boy," Marc said.

The dog emerged out of the darkness and sat right in front of me. It had an intensity in its eyes that I hadn't seen before. I turned around and began to walk in the same direction out of the cemetery.

Marc stepped in front of me and said, "We're going to finish what we started, you understand?"

Every muscle in my body tensed up in fear, but I squeezed out the last objection. "No, we really have to go," I said.

"No, not we. You mean *you* must go. And you can't go anywhere because I'm the muthaf***a with the car," he said.

"I can't..."

"Here's how this whole thing is going to go down, punk-ass faggot. You're going to suck my dick real good, pull down your pants and give me that ass you've been switchin' in my face all night. Period," he said.

I had two choices, fight or flee. I tried to judge in my head the distance from the center of the cemetery to Airport Road and whether I could run fast enough in the dark while navigating through a maze of tombstones and trees. He read my mind. He knew exactly what I was thinking.

"You don't wanna run. Because if you run, Baron here will chase you down, and rip your f**kin face off, bitch. So I wouldn't recommend that," he said.

The dog growled in my direction and showed all of its teeth.

"Marc, please!" I begged.

"Who's Marc?" he asked with a grin.

"Shit."

There was no way I could outrun a Doberman, so I did what any gay, black, skinny kid with a stutter would do in that situation. I punched that nigga square in his face and ran. I felt the teeth of his dog nipping at my calves and ankles, and then I was tackled to the ground, not by the dog, but by him.

I fought him off the best I could. He was definitely over six feet tall and easily weighed over 200 pounds. He had massive upper body strength, which he used to pummel my face, torso, and thighs with punches. At some point, I lost consciousness for a few seconds because, when I came to, my jeans were unfastened and pulled halfway down my thighs. My thighs were purple and black and numb with pain. I remember not being able to move them. And out of the corner of my eye, I saw a glimpse of moonlight reflect off the stainless-steel blade, seconds before I felt its cold, sharp edge against my throat. I froze as warm blood trickled down my face.

It's true what they say about near-death experiences. Everything unfolded in slow motion. The cold knife pierced my neck, just deep enough through the skin and tissue for me to stop fighting back. His erect penis rested right at the crack of my butt. I saw my life flash before my very eyes, like an old, black-and-white silent horror film. And just like one of those films, no one was coming to my rescue.

Tears mixed with blood from my busted nose and split lip ran down my chin. I saw an image of my Aunt Mary, far off, worried, and pale. She hadn't slept all night, wondering where I could be. I thought how much I loved my dear aunt who took me into her home and life and how sorry I was for not being what she, or anyone else, wanted. At that moment, that realization pained me more than anything I was experiencing during the rape. He spat on his penis to facilitate lubrication and violently penetrated me. He mushed my face into the stiff ground and cursed at me while he did it.

Ironically, the more he brutalized me, the less relevant the sex act seemed. As monstrous as he was, that individual became a minor character whose sole purpose was to reveal more profound truths about my existence. And I hated that revelation. I hated myself more and more with every thrust. I hated I was gay. I hated that the "curse" of my sexuality, and my weakness for a man's affection and validation, placed me in precarious situations – repeatedly. I was going nowhere fast, and I wanted off that merry-go-round called my life.

I was dizzy with self-deprecation and disdain. I prayed to God for forgiveness for my sins, but when he finished, a significant piece of James Ford never made it out of that cold dark cemetery that night. I lost him to it. It consumed him.

From the fragments of an abused James and remnants of an abandoned Jof, a year later, Jasmine would emerge – a personality steeped in strength, confidence, and control... or a personality particularly exceptional at feigning these qualities.

"Come on, let's walk to the car. It's cold as shit out here," he said.

I didn't look at him. I couldn't look at him. I put myself back together the best I could and walked a slight distance behind and to the left of him. Why did I get into the vehicle of a guy who had just beaten me up and raped me, many people often asked? The answer I gave was practical. I was scared, alone, and a long way from home. I sat within arm's reach from my rapist, on the passenger side, for what seemed to be an eternity. I was approximately 15 miles away from my home.

I remember looking out of the car window the entire ride. I mumbled directions to my rapist without ever glancing over in his direction. I was slightly comforted as I watched familiar street signs, buildings, and stores whiz by as the car traveled down Union Boulevard toward Bethlehem. It felt as though I was holding my breath until we came to the intersection of Main Street and Union Boulevard.

We caught the red light. The streets were bare, not a soul in sight. My heart pounded like a bass drum while my palms were drenched in sweat. I directed him to continue past the intersection for another block, where he could drop me off. I didn't want him to know where I lived. I pulled my swollen, sore body out of the car and watched him speed off.

When his taillights were only a blur in the distance, I ran yelling down the block to 803. By the time I crossed the Sunoco gas station and mini-mart, the lights in my house had come on in the front bedroom that faced the street. That was my Aunt Mary's bedroom. My entire body collapsed against the front door. I was out of breath and in a lot of pain. It felt as though I had run a marathon.

Crying and shaking, I knocked feverishly on the front door. Moments later, I saw her standing on the landing of the stairs. Aunt Mary opened the door, and from the way I looked, she knew exactly what had happened. It was two and a half hours past my curfew. She looked me up and down, from the crown of my head to the soles of my feet, and rushed me inside.

"Shhh! Don't come in here whooping, hollering and crying, and carrying on. You're gonna wake the whole house up. Go straight upstairs to the bathroom and run yourself a nice hot bath — as hot as you can stand

it. Aunt Mary is gonna fix you up, chile...
Lord have mercy," she whispered.

I limped past her, climbed the stairs,
and made my way to the bathroom. I sat
on the rounded rim of the pearl white
cast-iron bathtub, drew water as hot as I
could stand, undressed, and slowly lowered
myself in. The fresh wounds scattered over
my body stung as they met the scorching
water, which quickly became ensanguined as
my limbs relaxed and soaked.

"Are you in the tub? Cover up, I'm com-
ing in," she said.

She sat on the toilet less than two feet
away from me, reached into her housecoat,
and pulled out an old aluminum container
of ointment. I was a seventeen-year-old
young man, totally oblivious to my naked-
ness before my aunt. I sat expressionless
in her presence. Vacant. We remained in
silence for a few moments, opposite of one
another. The only sound between us was the
splash of water against my broken brown
skin.

"You know something, that hole in your
heart got you lookin' for love in all the
wrong places, and it's gonna be the death
of you, boy, and it scares me. You may not
want to hear it, but things like this will

always happen to people like you. It's not right, and it's not fair. That's just the way it is," she said.

Bitter tears sprang up from deep within me as I slowly drank in her horrifying declaration. My very soul knew it to be true, and it wept for me. But to hear those words leap out of the mouth of a woman I'd loved with all of my heart, on the most devastating night of my life, was absolutely gut-wrenching.

I never looked her in the eye. I was far too ashamed. Embarrassed. Instead, while she spoke, I busied myself by tracing the many cracks and lines on my shriveled fingertips with my eyes.

"I've known men who loved men and women who loved women all my life. The Bible says *there is nothing new under the sun.* I couldn't tell you where to find that verse in the Bible. Nobody in this house knows more about the word of God than you. Yet, here you are. Just think about that while you soak. And take a finger full of that salve on the sink and place it on the open sores you have. Now it's gonna sting, but it's gonna help you heal a lot faster."

I glanced over at the old, dented, greasy can of ointment. The label and directions were illegible, smudged, and faded.

"Thank you, Aunt Mary. Can you please turn the light out when you leave?" I said.

"No, I won't. What you're not gonna do is disappear in the dark. Do you think you're the only person who's made a terrible decision and found themselves face-to-face with a crazy-ass man? Huh? Well, you ain't. You're not the first, and you damn sure won't be the last. So shake that thought outta your head right now. I love you, Josh. I love you more than you know. And God knows I didn't take you in, scuffle to raise you, and then have to bury you before your eighteenth birthday. But that's the direction you're headed in. I'm old, sick, and set in my ways, and I ain't changing no time soon, but I know one thing for sure — it's not what you do, but how you do it. You've got a very vulnerable and fragile spirit. You always have. You're smart, foolish, and kind, all at the same time. And that's a dangerous combination. I reckon that the only thing worse than that would be if you were stupid, foolish, and kind. You are certainly your mother's child. Carla was also smart as a whip, foolish and kind, and life just ripped her to shreds and drove her crazy. And it will do the same to you if you aren't careful and If you aren't strong. You just can't be black, gay, and weak in this world and survive. You just can't. Josh, I realize now that some of the pain and longing you feel is partly my fault, and for that, I am deeply sorry. Did I want to take in two small children to raise? No, I did not. But after you got here, I come to love you just the same. I always knew you were different. Hell, even Ray Charles could see that. I should've told you more often that your uniqueness was your sweetness. Maybe you would not hate yourself so much. Understand what I'm telling you?" she said.

"The thing that hath been, it is that which shall be; and that which is done is that which shall be done: and there is no new thing under the sun," I said.

"What?"

"The Bible verse you referenced is Ecclesiastes 1:9," I said softly, over my shoulder, in the direction of the bathroom door. "And I love you too, Aunt Mary."

"Uh-huh! Smart, foolish, and kind. If I were you, kiddo, I'd work on the middle one," she said with a smile.

I spent the next day alone, in my attic bedroom. Through the labyrinth-like heating vents that ran throughout our old house, I heard my aunt confide to her son what had occurred in the early morning. There was no such thing as a private conversation when spoken within earshot of the vents. Tina and I knew that fact better than anyone. The best family gossip was always divulged in the kitchen; over time, we learned that slanting the blades that controlled the amount of heat that came into a room during the winter also amplified sound.

"Don't say a damn word, but Josh was raped somewhere in Allentown, early this morning. He came in the house all beat up and bloody. I just didn't know what to say or do for that child," she said.

"The little nigga got what? Raped? Who the f**k let themselves get raped? And by who?"

"I don't know, Rome."

And then he laughed. It was a big, bellowing, full-throated laugh. He laughed as though he was bursting at the seams. The sound of it was ghostly, cruel, and irreverent. My cousin laughed as though he knew I was listening. The rape took an enormous chunk out of my soul, and that horrific laugh devoured whatever was left. I felt defeated and angry.

I never called the police. I did not want to subject my family to any additional public ridicule or scrutiny because of my sexuality. I believe the best parts of my humanity were left behind to rot among the bony tombstones that night.

Bed of Lies

Eager fingers fondled the
switch,

and the crimson light cracked
the darkness,

and upstaged the arrogance of
an opaque sky.

The light made visible for
the very first time that eve,

the quaint charm of her
abode-

which smelled of lilies and
lilac.

On her bed of perfect
pleasure,

She waited patiently on the
promises from her pimp,

But until her shepherd
arrived, she was the red
light special.

Every night she brought the
noise to her ear,

To hear the serpents, hiss
their requests,

and proffer her full hips and
rosy lips.

    "A shilling for a kiss?"

    "A buck for a bang?"

With every new fingerprint
that tattooed her flesh,

With every hand that
negotiated her bones,

With every violent
introduction into her dark
wetness,

she laid exposed. More
convinced of her abandonment.

The power in his promise
slowly fizzled,

and the surety of her rescue
packed up and left,

and poached a portion of her
dignity and self-respect.

On her bed of perpetual
pleasure,

she entertained his lies of
love,

perched on her cozy cot of
contempt.

As the blaring beacon howled,
night after night,

Summoning her suitors, duty,
and obligation

gave way to desperation and
despair.

Every night she brought the
noise to her ear,

to hear the Demons, delight
in her demise

and proffered up to them her
fraught hips and sallow lips.

"A farthing for a kiss?"

"A piece of tin for a bang?"

Thoughts of his return now played on the tracks of her mind,

like an old, scratched vinyl record- off-beat and obsolete.

She laid prone on her bed of pitiful pleasure.

Her soured insides reeked of spoiled cabbage,

Salve and ointment.

Supple flesh ripe for the right price now wept with decay.

As she lay on her bed of perpetual persecution, bound and broken.

The spent whore cried out in tears of yearning, far beyond the crimson

> lit night, for God to make
> his power manifest, and end
> her insufferable plight.
>
> J.C. Ford

Section 4 (The Lady and the Pimp)

It was early 2004; I was at the height of
my "career" as an escort and enjoyed a
blossoming career as a telemetry nurse at
Cedars Medical Center in downtown Miami.
I truly loved using my newly developed
clinical judgment and bedside manner to
assist patients along the path to well-
ness. Becoming a nurse was one of the most
intellectually challenging and reward-
ing achievements of my life. Still, the
allure of high-end prostitution was far
more tantalizing.

I never considered the possibility that
my involvement in sex work stemmed from
unresolved trauma as a child, but viewed
it as merely a substantial financial means
to an end. By 2004, I was in the midst
of a very lucrative career in the adult
entertainment industry. I quickly rose the

ranks to become one of the most successful transgender escorts in Miami.

This was when social media was in its infancy, and pornography hadn't saturated the internet. Subscription websites were on the rise, and I leaped at an opportunity to launch Cheyennexxx.com, with me as the featured talent. The website charged $29.99 for a monthly membership and/or $5.00 to download a five-minute clip.

Around the same time, I infiltrated most of the high-end escort services in all the major markets- New York City, Connecticut, the Hamptons on Long Island, Philadelphia, Los Angeles, Miami, Boston, Chicago, Dallas, Washington, D.C., Las Vegas, Seattle, and Denver. I used the word "infiltrate" because high-end escort agencies weren't interested in working with transgender models or service providers. Transgender women, especially of color, weren't perceived as marketable, desirable, or in demand with the heterosexual clientele who patronized these services.

Owners of adult agencies soon realized, though, that I represented a previously untapped market. They hired me as a premier "unique" talent: Black, beautiful, sophisticated, well-spoken, with a desirable body and packing an immense surprise.

Like thousands of other transgender sex workers across the country, I owe my success to the clandestine sexual proclivity of the *down-low brotha'* and their affinity for beautiful women with penises. Between porn and prostitution, men from every race, religion, and socioeconomic strata who identify as heterosexual contributed generously to the multi-billion-dollar industry, within which I was a flaming success. I was making six figures, tax-free, by 2008.

I was a beautiful girl, but my claim to fame was my body. I stood 5'7", weighed 140 pounds, measured 36DD-22-46, and was well-endowed in my panties (if you know what I mean).

My physical attributes alone didn't make me a success; they merely brought the "boys to the yard." It was intellect, customer service skills, and integrity as a call girl that became my calling card. I know I just paired the words "integrity" and "call girl" in the same sentence, but let me explain my rationale.

A lifestyle was introduced to me inundated with illicit drug use, alcohol, and all other forms of debauchery. Clients, especially white clients, were drawn to the fact that they found a provider who was a nurse and did not drink alcohol, do drugs, curse, steal, or try to skimp on services. I was not in the business to extort money from married men; in fact, I was extremely discreet and would go to extreme lengths to protect my clients' identity. In many eyes, I was the safer choice.

This so-called "work ethic" garnered me VIP clients such as NBA players, actors, comedians, football players, R&B singers, rappers, and other celebrity personalities from New York to L.A. It was amid the outlandish lifestyle I was leading that I met the love of my life.

"Hey, Mrs. Cookie, can I borrow a couple hundred dollars? I'm short on my rent. I promise I will pay you back when I get back from seeing Tariq in L.A.," I said.

"Wait a minute, bitch. Did you just walk into my apartment, not even ask how my old ass was feeling, flop that big silicone-injected ass on my couch, and proceed to ask me for some money? Where they do that at, hoe?" Mrs. Cookie said.

"Mrs. Cookie, really? How are you, Mother Cookie? Was that better, Mrs. Thing?" I asked as I reached for a tangerine in the fruit bowl placed as a centerpiece on her coffee table.

"Jasmine, you know I love you. I have been your trans mother since you moved to Florida in your mid-twenties. You and I have been through some shit together. You and Nadia are my beautiful babies. That's why I feel that it is my right as your trans mother and friend to ask you a question that I already know the answers to. What the f**k are you doing with all the money you make nursing and tricking?" she said.

"Mrs. Cookie, if you love me like you constantly claim, then do me a favor and spare me your tired, unsolicited speech on trans relationships. Or at least, on my relationship," I responded, slowly peeling my tangerine.

"Oh no, little girl. You got this old queen twisted. You don't get to interrupt my *General Hospital*. Especially since I waited all year to find out that Cesar Faison is still alive posing as Duke. And I just have to find out what happened to the real Duke Lavery," she said.

"Cookie, are you going to lend me the money or not?" I interrupted.

"I'll tell you what, Jasmine, if I can't say my piece in my own house about my own money, then you can go back to your apartment. An apartment where rent is due, with nothing except for the lint in your pockets and that half-eaten tangerine. I don't mind loaning money, but it's the reason why you need money that got me so pissed off at you," Cookie said, as she took off her soap-opera-watching glasses.

"Why do you have such an issue with Tariq, Cookie?"

"Did your Aunt Mary body slam you on your head when you peed the bed as a child? The question is, you dumb bitch, why don't you have a problem with Tariq? As a matter of fact, let me count the many ways Tariq is a problem. I know all your tea, so you can't deny a damn thing I'm about to say," she said.

I wanted to punch that noisy bitch in her face so bad. But I needed the money. I didn't trust myself not to, so I sat on the couch with my arms tightly folded and my legs crossed as she proceeded to go in on me. And when Cookie went in, she didn't pussy-foot around; that old bag of wrinkles went off.

"Girl, you know Mrs. Cook ain't a delicate queen. I never gave a shit about what a muthaf**** thought about me. There is no easy way to say this, so I'm gonna come right out and say it. Because all the math adds up… This man is pimping you, you special needs black bitch. What disturbs me is that I have watched you sit at my kitchen table studying psychology, biology, genetics, and all kinds of other bullshit for eight to 10 hours straight. I have cooked dinner for you and your brother Michael while you wrote twelve- and fourteen-page papers. And it baffles me that you can't read the writing on the wall of your own relationship. And I bet you I can back up anything I just said. Who pays Tariq's rent and brand new car note?"

"I do," I said solemnly through pursed lips as I shifted my position.

"And because you're transgender, you're not even permitted to visit him at the condo that you pay for every month, with money you earned on your back," Cookie said. Tears welled in the deep creases of her eyes, and her already husky voice began to break. I quickly averted my eyes from hers as she continued. Her voice ebbed and flowed with emotion. My gaze fell upon two miniature dogs that were commingled and asleep on the loveseat next to the couch.

"Why do we do this to ourselves, Jasmine? If someone such as yourself, possessing the privilege that comes with having beauty, body, and brains, can't escape the snares associated with a transgender identity, what hope do others have who don't?"

"Wow! Mrs. Cookie, you've been reading more than just the little letters in your cereal, I see. That mundane monologue brimming with self-indulgence and lunacy won't be nominated for any awards this season, I'm afraid. That category is closed. And furthermore, I never asked to be the spokesperson for my community anyway," I retorted.

"Well, if it's any consolation, you look fabulous today, as usual, Mrs. Jasmine," Mother Cookie said.

"You should have led with that," I said with a slight smile.

She reached into her purse beside her, counted out six hundred dollars in large bills, placed the wad of money in the palm of my left hand, and closed it.

Cookie walked me to the front door and opened it. She looked over the cars parked at the curb and stared at the beautiful Miami Beach skyline for a moment.

"I apologize, Jasmine. You're thirty-nine years old, and you're gonna do whatever you want to do in your relationship. And I respect that. However, my prayer is that you will have the courage to take off those technicolor glasses that you wear as protection one day soon. The world isn't as scary and cold as you have been made to believe, even for people like us," she said.

"No apology necessary, boo. I was always taught never to squabble with our senior citizens. Besides, I came to the conclusion eons ago that your crazy ass must be bipolar or something," I said.

I slowly sashayed down the stairs of her apartment and never looked back. It made the whole exchange shadier that way.

"You chicken-headed bitch," she yelled in my direction.

I quickly made a right onto Byron Avenue and 87th Street. The coast was clear. I was out of Mrs. Cookie's sight and finally felt safe enough to do what I had been dying to do ever since I graced her doorstep earlier that morning. I cried. And not your run-of-the-mill waterworks, either. Tears just didn't lazily ooze out of my ducts as I walked south on Byron toward my apartment on 81st. Tears erupted so forcefully from my eyes, my vision was blurred for the rest of the walk. It was an ugly, Celie from *The Color Purple* kind of cry. Why? Because sometimes the truth hurts, no matter who delivers it. And when in your most vulnerable moments, someone holds up to your face the mirror of truth, it eviscerates you. Occasionally, for your own good.

The fact of the matter was that I was in a relationship with an individual I loved far more than I loved myself. And I empowered him overtime to take control of my finances and escort service. My friends and family thought they knew everything about my relationship with Tariq, enough to formulate clever little jokes, jabs, and reads. But what I held close to the vest was that I gave that man over 90% of everything I earned throughout our four-year relationship. Which came to a total of $300,000.

The conversation I had with Mrs. Cookie, though crass in nature, was the impetus I needed to reexamine that relationship. And I broke up with Tariq. He was a down-low brother who had no intentions of existing openly with me. It turned out that our relationship meant very little to him, and I was merely a great source of income. I never retrieved a single penny of my money that was so-called invested in our future.

Don't feel sorry for me. Take heart: how I got it, was how I lost it.

Staring into the rearview mirror at one's life, things become very clear. As I began to categorize and prioritize my memories over these many years for my book, a few interesting themes emerged that I hadn't been consciously aware of in the past. And they posed more questions than answers. What I can say with a great sense of assurance is that I have gone to the extreme and, at times, extravagant lengths to hear the four-letter word embedded in an eight-letter phrase: "I love you."

In my mind's eye, I often found myself on the cold, soggy bands of unrequited love. In a cinched waist, I looked to the other side where such was lavishly plentiful, seething with envy.

What Church Is and Ought Not Be

Church ought not be
pretentious and puffed up
like a caged peacock —

inflated and proud, yet
tethered to the ground.

But Church is the place where
I can uproot my woes by the
bushel load,

And tote them on the broad of
my back, like a sack-a sweet
'tatoes.

Church ought not be a
collection of stiff-neck'd old
bones and dead souls,

Disguised in starched shirts,
petticoats, and choir robes.

But reverence for the
powerful preeminence of HIM,

Who indulges the foolery of
the absurd dreamer, and

Releases the hilariously
healed before us.

Church ought not be an
orchestra of lustful lurid
looks, bursting from blood-
shot eyes,

Cloaked behind flapping
faux lashes or penciled-in
mustaches.

But grant vision to us,
Oh Lord, that will barrel
through the heavens

Like an angry skyscraper.
Make manifest thy will, like
doodle with crayon

On a child's homework paper.

Church ought not be an
assemblage of the simple,
a colorful collage of the
unconscious,

Or a fanciful foyer for the
forlorn. Pacifying those who
have no intention of ever
being reborn.

But harken to the Seer of
the House, wide-winged and
balanced, high upon his
perch.

The gentle, omniscient
protector of all the earth.

"Hark! Hark!" the Eagle
blares.

"Write the vision, make
it plain, encourage your
brethren to do the same!"

"Perfect your vision, in
my name, *fratres vestri
auxilium*, so they too can
obtain!"

Church ought be like a gaggle
of galloping guppies; too
busy about HIS business to be
bothered,

Too secure in their
conviction to be scattered,
and too on task, for anything
else to matter.

I wish Church was...

J.C. Ford

Section 5 (Church Hurt: You Can't Sing in the Choir)

I had been a member of New Birth Baptist Church Cathedral of Faith International for a few years before I decided – or more accurately, was encouraged to join the choir. I was a faithful churchgoer who was hard-pressed to attend every worship service, whether in town or out. The Lord had begun to move heavily in my life. The Holy Spirit was helping me deal with a lot of the trauma I had suffered, and so I pursued the word of God like a crackhead chases after crack. I had found love again, but this time it had absolutely nothing to do with the flesh.

Every Sunday, a service servant leader would get up on the pulpit and remind parishioners that it was their duty as children of God to utilize the spiritual gifts divinely bestowed by the Father for the church's benefit and to the glory of God. So three members of the "clan" joined the church's mass choir.

Raquel (my best friend at the time), Sir Diego, and I all showed up at the next choir rehearsal. The choir was scheduled to honor their old director, who had been retired quite some time, the following

Sunday. I was excited, but that excitement would be only temporary.

New Birth Baptist Church in Miami is a relatively large worship center. I was filled with awe as I walked down the center aisle that Saturday morning. I stepped onto the altar and then onto the massive choir stand that majestically overlooked the sanctuary. I felt proud and blessed to be a part of such a wonderful, progressive ministry.

I sat with the sopranos. Raquel and Sir Diego, who each had a significant amount of vocal ability, were placed with the tenors for the first rehearsal. When I sat down in my section, most choir members gave me hugs and were very welcoming; however, others sneered, pointed, and whispered among themselves. That behavior from the gallery of haters and church spectators, I honestly expected. I got that every Sunday from the usual suspects. But what I did not expect, and crept up on me like a "thief in the night," happened later that evening.

After the rehearsal, Diego slid over to speak to Jose, the Pastor of Music and Arts, while Raquel and I left. Later that evening, Raquel came over to my condo on

79th and Collins Avenue on Miami Beach with an overnight bag that carried her church clothes. Raquel was a cisgendered (biological) female, thirteen years my senior, who was my very best friend; I trusted her with everything. Although she was not transgender, we related to one another like sisters.

Raquel often communicated to me that she was a heterosexual woman with a spectrum. Which, in layman's terms, simply meant that she was a freak. She was my biggest cheerleader, and I hers. Raquel's place was the usual hub for the clan to hang out after church, where we would eat, chit-chat, debate about life's issues (which often turned into love-filled but heated arguments), and just enjoy the wonderful friendship we had discovered.

It was around 7:30 PM. I made my Aunt Mary's famous smothered pork chops, fried cabbage with salted pork, and baked macaroni and cheese. This dish was Raquel's favorite, and I would prepare it for her or the entire clan on special occasions such as holidays or birthdays. And this qualified, because the next day, we would be singing in front of the whole church: an openly transgender woman, an openly gay man, and our sidekick ally with the spectrum.

I was still putting the finishing touches on the meal when my cell phone rang. The the conversation went something like this.

"Hello, Jasmine. This is Elder Whitehead. Do you have a few moments to speak with me?"

Elder Whitehead was the Executive Pastor of New Birth Baptist Church. It was highly uncommon for me to receive a call from anyone in leadership at that level. I repeated her name out loud, and Raquel stopped eating and sat next to me on the couch.

"Yes, of course, Pastor Whitehead. I can talk. Is anything wrong?" I asked.

"I understand that you were over at the church earlier today to join the choir. Is that correct, Jasmine?" she asked.

"Yes, ma'am. A few of us decided to join the mature choir because it would allow us to serve and not commit ourselves to sing almost every Sunday like the mass choir."

And then it happened. The conversation I vowed to myself that I would never ever have with a senior member of any church body. Why? Because I wouldn't be foolish enough as a transgender woman to put myself in the position to be hurt.

I was bamboozled. I joined a ministry a few years earlier. After much priming, I believed their slogan that, "New Birth is the perfect place for imperfect people." I thought I, like everyone else, was a sinner who was saved by grace. I believed in my heart all saints not only have read the entire book of Ephesians but committed it to heart.

"You know that we love you here at New Birth, and it breaks my heart have to tell you this because you have confided in me some of the things you have been through. Jasmine, you cannot be in the choir. Some people believe and have brought it up to Bishop Curry that an individual born male, and transitioned into a female, should not be on the pulpit or in the choir stand behind the Bishop. I have spoken on your behalf, but the board stated that sort of thing wouldn't go over well with the congregation. I'm sorry. I genuinely hope that this doesn't negatively affect your spiritual walk with Christ. I have watched you come out of your shell, so I hope this situation doesn't shut you back off. You are graciously welcomed to worship with us every Sunday as you usually do," she said.

As Pastor Whitehead delivered what sounded like an uncomfortable and well-rehearsed one-sided conversation, tears rolled down my face. Raquel looked on in shock and horror. "Please tell me they didn't do that to you, Jasmine. Oh, my God. Those hypocritical muthaf***as," Raquel yelled.

I just sat cross-legged on my couch and stared at the wall while Raquel called everyone in the 305 area code. Everyone in the clan wanted me to handle the situation more militantly than I was prepared to do. Diego believed that denying a transgender individual the opportunity to sing in a choir when one's ability to sing was not a factor was discrimination. His persistent advice to me was to go straight to the media and essentially take my story public and let the chips fall where they may.

Raquel and her transgender brother, Renee, suggested that I request a meeting with Bishop Curry and demand to know what biblical precept governed that decision. Because I knew for a fact that there were several open and closeted homosexual choir members, deacons, and other staff members.

During that period, many of those individuals expressed concern over how I would handle being slighted by the church. "Mrs. Jasmine, girl, I just heard about what happened. Chile, New Birth just ain't ready," Deacon A said.

"I honestly thought I had found a church that I could grow and serve in. I was expecting some pushback from certain individuals who openly hate me. Still, the bishop siding with this decision without a follow-up conversation with me is overwhelming," I said.

"I've been a deacon at New Birth for many years, and I have not seen anything like you grace those doors. Every Sunday, women break their necks to see what Jasmine is wearing. And you don't disappoint. Sis got on a brand new designer dress, shoes, hat, and handbag, looking more fish than these tired females. They absolutely did not want you and all that body in the choir stand. Between you and me, that decision had absolutely nothing to do with the Bible and everything to do with fear, tithes, and offerings. Because if membership in the choir was contingent upon one's lifestyle being 100% biblically sound, we wouldn't have a choir — at least not a good one. There are sissies, drug addicts, liars, whores, and thieves singing behind the Bishop every Sunday. And those are the ones I personally know of just in the tenor and alto section, respectfully. Females have children out of wedlock with individuals who have important positions in the church. They tell a transwoman who actually wants to serve that she cannot. Every Sunday, a different servant leader gets up in the pulpit and advertises various ministries, requesting church participation," Deacon B said.

"Exactly, and those are the people who should be coming to Christ, and we're not knocking them. And you know I know who you're talking about, by the way. But to exclude a transwoman when your choir is a cesspool of sin, really?" Deacon A said.

I listened to many opinions surrounding the choir fiasco. Still, I chose to pay closer attention to the Holy Spirit during my prayer time. I was instructed to stand firmly on my faith. So I continued to attend the same church, praise, and worship my God. I needed to demonstrate through my non-action a better example of God's grace, mercy, and love in the face of unspeakable church hurt and rejection. A decision truly easier said than done.

Section 6 (The Twisted Love of a Father)

It was 1990, and I was a high school senior, already committed to attend Miss Wade's Fashion Merchandising College in Dallas, Texas, the following June. Wade College (as it was renamed in 1999) offered me a partial scholarship in their Fashion Design program. And I could not have been more thrilled.

I was a well-rounded student with good grades. I had submitted a portfolio of my best, most innovative designs for consideration for admission. I was accepted within weeks after their deadline. Although I decided not to pursue a degree in psychology initially, my mother and Aunt Mary couldn't have been happier or more supportive.

On the outside, I was like all of my other high school friends. I had challenged myself academically all through my matriculation to get into college, and would soon reap the benefits of four years of hard labor. But inside, I was unlike anyone I knew. I had been silently dealing with my gender identity and the fear and confusion it caused me throughout my adolescence. It simply wasn't enough that I was a male who was attracted to and had intimate relationships with other males. There was a missing piece to the puzzle that initially I couldn't put my finger on in my youth. However, like a camera lens slowly coming into focus from ten to sixteen, it occurred to me.

I yearned to be in the body of a girl. This realization was evident on a subconscious level. When I discovered masturbation, like every other healthy kid does, I was a pretty girl in my fantasy. I was never a male. If my memory serves me correctly, I didn't identify as what society would label as transgender. I was not a girl with a penis in these daydreams or fantasies, nor a girl who had ever had a penis. I was just a girl.

My father and I had a relatively new relationship, that began when I was fourteen years old. He was married and fathered four children within his marriage and several more outside of it. This was an open secret that my father touted like a depraved badge of honor.

Early on, I enjoyed getting to know my biological father and the family he presented to me. At fourteen, I met a brother who was one year older than I was, whom I absolutely admired and adored, and several sisters who quickly captured my heart, and a stepmother who treated me as if I was one of her own, from day one.

In laying out the background in such a thorough manner, one can understand the relationships at risk if I told my father that I was strongly considering transitioning to female. My father was a pretty prominent boxer in the South Philadelphia area at the time, so I had prepared myself for a hyper-masculine, biblical rebuke of my transition. But instead, this is a rough account of how that very disturbing exchange unfolded.

I had left a message with his wife that I needed to speak with my father when he became available. He had gotten into the habit of checking in on me with the occasional phone call. I was living in Bethlehem while he still resided in South Philly with his family.

The day started like any other unremarkable Saturday in February. But this was the day that I mustered up the nerve to have a talk with him. My mother and Aunt Mary were upstairs, straightening up the front bedroom where my sister and aunt slept. I was downstairs alone, watching television in the middle room when the phone rang. I suspected it was my dad, so I quickly ran to the kitchen and grabbed the receiver off of the wall. I'm going to reproduce the conversation we had as though neither of us had a significant speech impediment, so feel free to use your imagination.

"Hello, Dad," I said.

"Hello, son. What's going on? I heard you wanted to talk to me," my father said.

Now that he was on the phone and was hanging onto my every word, I got cold feet. I beat around the bush for several moments more until he said, "Jof, you know that you can tell Daddy anything. You can tell me anything, and I will still love you the same. You are my second-born baby boy."

My stomach felt like it was literally twisted in a series of knots. "I'm not happy as a boy, Daddy, and I am considering changing into a girl. They can do that kind of thing now, and I just wanted to know how you would feel about me doing that?"

"Wow! That's heavy. That's deep. That's deep, son. So let me get this straight. Doctors can make you into a woman with a real working vagina?" he asked.

"Yes, I guess so," I responded tentatively.

Then, after a moment, the conversation between my father and me took on an uncomfortable tone. Bizarre, actually, even for this subject matter.

"Well, I mean, if that's what you want to do, you'll be an adult. And let me educate you a little about men. You will have a new body with the hormones you just told me about and the surgery that will give you a vagina. Most men are not going to be gentle with you for your first time. They're going to rush and hurt you. And your first time having intercourse as a woman should be memorable," he said in a low tone.

And then, suddenly, the words fell out of his mouth in almost a stuttering whisper. "Do you think Daddy could be the first to penetrate you? Be your first experience after you've had the surgery?" my father asked.

My memory of this conversation is still fresh, vivid, and palpable, even after 32 years.

I didn't say a word for the first few seconds. I waited for a punch line. But, there was no punch line. I took the phone away from my ear, held it in front of my face, and just stared at it in utter shock.

I needed immediate assurance that I hadn't gone completely crazy. Did I actually hear what I had heard? Or was I reading too much into an awkward conversation about sex changes, and my paranoia had reached an all-time high? I needed confirmation of either.

"Daddy, I heard only some of the conversation. Our phone has been acting up. But from what I did hear, sounds interesting. Hang on, so I can fix the phone, and we can continue the conversation. I'm so relieved you are so supportive," I said.

I put the phone down gently and ran upstairs to the front bedroom where my mother and aunt were talking. "Mom! Aunt Mary!" I shouted as I slid into her bedroom. "Something strange just happened. Please don't yell, and please don't scream. But I'm pretty sure that my dad just came on to me over the phone," I stuttered.

"*What?*" Aunt Mary said.

"Is he still on the phone?" my mother asked.

"Yes, I got him on hold. I told him the phone was acting up. I don't know what to say," I said.

"Quickly and quietly lift up that receiver, and hand it to me, Jof. And run back downstairs and continue that conversation like nothing is wrong. I need to hear what that crazy Negro is talking about to my child," my mother commanded.

When I left the room, each of them had an ear to the receiver. I ran back downstairs and resumed the conversation.

"I'm sorry for the wait, Daddy, but I can hear you clearer now. Can you repeat the last part of what you were saying? You were giving me advice about sex after my surgery," I said.

My father repeated himself practically verbatim.

My mother appeared out of nowhere, with our aunt right behind her. Once they heard what they needed to hear, they must have literally jumped down a flight of stairs. My aunt had a history of leg pain and often carried a cane. But that day, she moved like Jackie Joyner-Kersee. Aunt Mary snatched the phone out of my hand and screamed.

"Hello, Keith? This is Aunt Mary. I just heard the filth you just said to your son. This boy is having a hard time. He is thinking about changing his whole life with surgery. Because he is so lost and confused, and unhappy, and he wanted to reach out to his father for advice. And this is how you do your child? Let me tell you one muthaf**king thing, you nasty bastard. If you ever call my house looking for Josh, you're gonna have to deal with my son," she said.

My mother took her turn. She grabbed the phone from Aunt Mary and released a barrage of profanity too explicit even for this book. But you get the idea. They were pretty upset.

That incident, I dare say, single-handedly destroyed my perception of what a healthy father-child relationship should look like — forever. It further contorted my sense of identity, as male or female, and gutted my already low opinion of men. I had prepared myself for virtually any other response except the one he gave. I could have psychologically reconciled any other reaction from a "saved man of God."

My father and I did not speak to one another for quite a while. Our relationship was irretrievably fractured, or so I thought. I continued on that year to graduate from Liberty High School. A year later, I began my gender transition, relocated back to Philadelphia a few years after that, and subsequently planted roots in Miami, Florida, all without hearing a single word from my father.

When I was twenty-seven years old, I received a phone call from my older brother Kenny. He informed me that our father had been arrested and indicted for sexually abusing one of our younger siblings. During his trial, it was revealed that he had been molesting a few of his children over many years. He was subsequently convicted and would spend more than thirteen years in prison.

Section 7 (The Twisted Love of a Father, Part 2)

It was 2012, and I had faithfully attended New Birth Baptist Church every Sunday for the past two years. It was at New Birth where I met my circle of friends, affectionately called the clan. We were a band of churchgoing misfits, according to the judgmental eyes that fell on us each week, whom I came to adore.

Although I was still working as a call girl, I began to develop a conscience about how I made money, which I relieved through my frequent church attendance and the Holy Spirit. It was during this precious time of rededication to Christ and tremendous spiritual growth that I began to slowly open up my heart, which had been closed for so many years.

I was about forty years old when my father was finally released from prison. I was informed of his release by one of my many siblings he had created outside of his marriage. During my father's stint in prison, something miraculous occurred between the twenty-two children he left behind thirteen years earlier. We made a concerted effort to meet one another, if we hadn't already done so. Facebook was an incredible resource.

The full siblings were understandably closer than half-siblings. Regardless, we understood the importance of coming together, if only for the benefit of collective healing from the trauma sustained at the hands of an absent, abusive father. So, in the spirit of healing and moving forward in life, I learned that some of my brothers and sisters were planning on throwing our father a welcome home party in Philadelphia.

Initially, honestly, I thought they were crazy. But the more I was exposed to the reason behind the grand gesture, I concluded that their intentions were heroic and nothing short of Godly. I was the second-oldest, and I was admittedly a little envious of the amount of maturity and grace my younger siblings displayed toward our father.

I also wanted to experience that level of healing and forgiveness after so many years. The more I pondered the possibility, the more my heart needed it. I agreed that I would attempt to have a relationship with my father if he took the initiative to first reach out to me in Miami.

After the big shindig was thrown in his honor and he got settled into his new life as a free man, my father called me.

Our initial conversation was a very odd one. I was approaching forty years old and hadn't heard my father's voice in decades. I had developed externally into the woman

I had described feeling like internally so many years earlier. Some of that conversation went like this.

"Hello, can I please speak to Jof?" my father said.

"Hi, Daddy. This is Jasmine. My name is Jasmine now, Daddy," I replied.

"Oh! Is this really you? You sound just like a woman. Wow! Wow! Wow!" he said. "So, you're a woman now?" he asked.

"Yes, and have been for quite some time. How are you? I heard everyone threw you a big party a few weeks ago. How was that?" I said.

"Aw man, it was beautiful. Your sisters Kee Kee and Nadine mostly organized it. Many of your brothers and sisters were there. Why didn't you come?"

"I honestly didn't know whether I was invited or even if I wanted to be there," I said.

"Well, I'm calling you because I wanted to tell you that I am sorry for any pain I have caused you, and if you allow me, I want to get to know my daughter Jasmine. Being away gave me a lot of time to think about my actions and how my actions hurt my children. And just like I told the rest of them, I am asking for the opportunity to be in your life again. I already asked and received forgiveness from God. Now, I am asking for forgiveness from you," my father said.

My face was saturated with tears. I couldn't believe that the man on the other end of the phone was actually my dad. This man was open, kind, remorseful, intentional about the pronouns he used, and eager to know his adult transgender daughter. In those moments, it felt as though I had won the lottery. I couldn;t help but wonder if the Lord wa granting me the closure that I needed, with the love, attention, and approval from a father I desperately desired. My life appeared to finally be leveling out.

That first conversation sparked many more in the coming days, weeks, and months. My Father and I spoke often and about everything. I was attending Florida International University, where I was pursuing my degree in Interdisciplinary Studies with a minor in Psychology.

My mother, who had suffered an acute stroke twenty years earlier, became too ill for me to care for and had been placed in a nursing and rehabilitation center. She had been convalescing at the facility for about five years before my Father came back into my life. I saw her faithfully every Sunday after church, during weekday evening services, and whenever she needed me. I absolutely adored my mother, and she loved me right back- maybe not as much as she loved Coca-Cola and cigarettes. But, I came in a solid second to the pair. One afternoon during my visit after church service, In her failing health, my mother spoke ominously about the new relation- ship I had cultivated with my Father over the past year. I asked my mother not to be bitter or resentful. I told her that I believed in my heart that miraculous- ly, prison and prayer had changed him. He was no longer the man that she loathed in their youth.

"Jasmine, my baby. My oldest baby. You're beautiful and smart, but at the age of for- ty years old, you are still foolish. This man has identified what your heart lacks. What your heart has always lacked, and he has latched on to it. For what I reason, I do not know. But the sense of safety and security this man is creating between you and him is a smokescreen. The time this man devotes to you on the phone, giving decades late fatherly advice feels good, but it's not free," my mother said.

I sat on her bed and listened intently to my sweet mother's words of wisdom. I didn't say a word. I just held her hand and gave her my undivided attention. Mother knew me well. I needed to believe my Father more than I wanted to believe my mother. She spoke her peace and never broached the subject of my Father ever again.

Later, she and I would enjoy months of visits and outings filled with love, laughter, and light — until we finally ran out.

Carla Ester Ford died on May 23rd, 2013. She transitioned in my arms in the Intensive Care Unit at the University of Miami Hospital, where I was formerly employed as a nurse. My mother was fifty-nine years old. To state that I took my mother's death hard would be a profound understatement. I was emotionally and psychologically utterly unprepared for the process I had to go through. I didn't think that the human soul could grieve so deeply and survive. I found myself free-falling in a bottomless abyss of grief and despair. My only refuge was within the safety of the sanctuary. I would wail in the pews until I hyperventilated and nearly lose consciousness. I literally thought that I was going to die of a broken heart. I lost the unconditional love of a mother who has the unique ability to rebuke and affirm to stretch her offspring's potential beyond anyone's expectations. My mother's good pleasure was to give up her last so her children could have. And in the case of our mother, who loved her children earnestly through a disorganized, and often, overly medicated mind. I realized early in life how truly blessed my sister, and I was to have Carla as a mother. I am not a psychiatrist by any stretch of the imagination, but I associate Schizophrenia as a damp shroud of disorganized neural connections in the brain that tug at the fabric of one's sanity a little each day. My mother lived and loved through that haze as best as she could. We, I primarily, benefited tremendously from her sacrifice.

I obviously turned to rely heavily on my father for his love and support during the most devastating time of my life. I felt closer to him than I had ever had in my entire life. He became the father I never had. My dad even started giving me advice about faith, relationships, and dating. I felt attached and secure. So much so, I had forgotten the advice my mother gave me regarding my Father. The day he came to collect, I was at my lowest.

"Hello, my beautiful daughter," he began the conversation.

"I'm well, daddy, and you?" I said.

"Daddy is not doing well, and I think you are the only one who could make me feel better. I have seen all of your good girl pictures, with all of your clothes on. How about sending daddy some photos without?" he said.

At the time of this phone conversation, my father had recently buried his wife, Ethel. A woman who loved me like I was her own since I was thirteen years old.

I absolutely don't know what happened, but I found myself exchanging my escort photos with my Father. Grant it, I thought it was weird and inappropriate. But I was also a prostitute who blurred the lines of morality daily as a professional courtesy.

Over time our relationship degraded as Father and daughter. He begged me to fly to Philadelphia, pick him up, so we could get a hotel. He wanted us to spend the weekend together.

I remember being heartbroken and feeling utterly lost emotionally, psychologically, and spiritually. I thought, how did I get here?

I flew into Philadelphia airport and acquired a rental. The second he realized I had landed in town, my own Father blew my phone up like a desperate client. And I had a moment of clarity in front of my cousin Kay Kay's house in southwest Philadelphia. I sat outside in my rental, shaking and crying in disbelief at myself.

And the Holy Spirit comforted me and provided me the clarity that I needed.

I didn't feel like myself because I wasn't myself. I was in the body of forty-year-old Jasmine, but it was little six-year-old Jof who would do anything for a father's love. I gave my body away for money to complete strangers. And in my warped reality at the time, I might be willing to do one despicable act for lasting love. I wept for little Jof even more. My phone had 45 missed calls and text messages from him. I turned my cell phone off, cleaned my face up with some eyeliner, and walked into my Aunt Missy's house. She was one of my Father's sisters and the mother of my favorite outrageous first cousin Kay Kay.

"Hey, baby," Aunt Missy said with a broad smile sitting on the couch.

"Hello, Aunt Missy," I said, as I gave her a hug.

She looked me dead in the eyes and saw something that prompted her to ask, "Spoke to your father lately?"

"Yes, we speak," I said.

"Why are you in Philadephia, Jasmine? It seems like you were just here hanging out with Kay Kay a few weeks ago," she said.

"I don't know. I guess I miss it so much," I said.

"My spirit is telling me something is not quite right with you, but I'm gonna trust that you're gonna tell your Aunt Missy when you're ready. Go in the kitchen and make yourself a plate. Aunt Missy made some fried chicken," she said.

"Yes, ma'am," I said.

"Are you staying the night, or are you getting a hotel like you usually do?" Aunt Missy asked.

"If you don't mind, Aunt Missy, I would like to spend the night on the couch, if you don't mind," I said.

"Stop it. You know you are welcome here in my home anytime for as long as you like. Eat and get some rest, pretty girl," she said.

I tucked my cell phone into my purse. I ate like a pig. And Kay Kay and I talked and threw shade at each other well into the night. Which was and is our language of love. I later got sheets and covers for the couch and slept like a well-fed six-year-old.

My Aunt Missy patched a leaking heart with fried chicken made with unconditional love. The kind of love that doesn't come to collect. That night, unbeknownst to her, she became one of the most recent super-women applied to my life.

I never spoke to my father ever again.

Chapter 5: Tricks and Trade

Section 1 (The Rapper and the Extreme Case of Buyer's Remorse)

"Hello. Can I please speak to Cheyenne?" a man asked.

"This is she. Who's calling?"

"I got your number from another colleague in the industry, and he said that you are beautiful, safe, and very discreet to your VIP clientele," he said.

"What industry is that?"

"The music industry," he replied.

"Oh, okay! Great! How can I help you?"

"I actually can't believe that I am calling somebody like you for services, but I am looking to have my first experience with a female like you today. I'm a rap artist, in town to present at the Source Awards tonight. So you tell me what I need to do to make this happen because I'm nervous and scared as f*ck," he said.

When speaking to rich, famous clients, my business practice was to communicate with them in a low, calm voice. I never appeared excited to hear from them, nor did I ask them for any identifying information. Why not? Because I didn't give a crap.

"Calm down, sweetheart. Your associate steered you in the right direction. I can arrive when you need me to and leave only when you are deliciously satisfied. My rate for VIP clients is $700 per hour, with a two-hour minimum. I provide a full, intimate girlfriend experience. And how intimate we get during the girlfriend experience honestly depends on what you look like and not how much you spend. Foremost, I am a safety girl. I *always* use condoms, so don't ask me if you can go raw because the answer will be a resounding *hell no*. I communicate to new clients my dos and don'ts just to limit any confusion when we link up. And finally, how would you like me to dress coming to your hotel?"

"All that you just said sounds cool. Just come looking sexy and girlie. I'm at the Delano Hotel on South Beach. Are you familiar with the hotel?"

"I've been in every hotel worth staying in, from Miami to West Palm Beach," I said with a laugh.

"Damn! For real," he said.

I dressed sexy yet appropriate for an afternoon romp on South Beach. I wore a skin-tight dress, showing oodles of curves, and my sun-kissed face was dusted lightly with makeup.

Once I reached his hotel room door, I quickly put on my *"nigga, I'm not impressed that you're a rapper"* face, readjusted my breasts in my dress, and knocked on the door. I recognized him immediately from his music videos and many television appearances.

"Hello, I'm Cheyenne."

"Hey sweetheart, come on in. Wow! You look better than what my homeboy said," he said.

I knew his hit rap song, which was in constant rotation on the radio station 99 JAMS in Miami. This man was super fine, tall, and was living in the skin color that made my hair weave stand on end.

Once he let me in the room and got the pleasantries out of the way, I began the session like I routinely did. "That will be $1,400, sweetheart. Cash or charge?" I said.

"Bet! What do I get for $3,000?" he said.

This Negro was seriously talking my love language now. I don't care how rich, famous, or hung a man is: money talks and bullshit walks. "Sweetheart, for $3,000, I'll have you in here purring like a cat in heat. I might even grow a uterus, bear down, grunt, and deliver to you a bouncing baby boy — complete with his own hit nursery rhyme," I said as I snaked my way from the foot of the bed to the headboard.

"Naw, I'm cool on the baby tip. That's part of the reason I'm here with a trans," he said as he lit a blunt.

I had intentionally slipped in a feminine metaphor to feel him out. I wanted to see what I was really working with behind closed doors.

"So this will be completely confidential, right? I got a lot to lose. And your name came highly recommended by some top individuals in my industry. And I am curious about…" he asked.

"Curious about what?" I repeated as I squirmed on the king-size bed in anticipation of his answer. I knew what it was. I knew who he was. And before my very eyes, he shed that expensive facade of hyper-masculine, rapper mentality bullshit like a snake sheds its skin. He dropped to his knees before me, reached his hand under my dress until he found what he'd been secretly yearning for for most of his life.

My escort character Cheyenne knew how to draw men out of their comfort zone in a beautifully engaging way. They paid me to create a world within a world, for 60 minutes at a time. I was their puppet master, fashioned in Cartier jewels, stiletto heels, and the finest collection of corsets my money could buy. My clients could be anyone or anything they wanted, and I never judged them. Well, at least never to their faces. Over time, this became a well-crafted talent and an occupational hazard. It was the reason I could command so much money and get it, too.

"I want us both to give each other head, and I want us to f**k each other," the rapper guy said.

Ding. Ding. Ding. And the lady gets a prize. I do not intend to provide explicit details about my old profession. I merely want to give the reader a glimpse into some experiences that helped shape who I was during that period in my life, which informed any decisions I subsequently made.

I will say for the sake of discretion that this famous client was in the mood to experiment, and I obliged his every whim. He was an excellent time…until.

"Shit, Cheyenne, I can't believe I let you do that bullshit to me," he growled as he got dressed.

Admittedly, the session had gotten very heated. We were having sex like we were a couple for real. I was more intimate with the rapper guy than I usually allowed myself to get with any other client. He was rich, black, and famous, and hung like a horse.

I have discovered through my transition that the relationship between men and transgender women is precarious. Men like him are trying to filter through a rush of emotional information. Trans-attracted men first address their internal desire to be with a transgender woman, in whatever capacity. Case in point: the entertainer sought the services of a transgender sex worker to satisfy a fantasy that had probably been secretly brewing for quite some time, and masturbation was no longer sufficient.

Second, these men continually survey what society says regarding sexuality. Usually, this messaging is negative, homophobic, and transphobic. We met discreetly in a luxury hotel on South Beach during a scheduled work-related engagement in a city he did not live in. I certainly was not invited to the Source Awards as his date. I would never have been welcome on his arm in public, whether I *passed* as a cisgender female or not.

Third, it forces these men to evaluate themselves, and their sexual behavior, through a social lens that assigns them the new pejorative title of homosexual or bisexual. As his hormones leveled out immediately after he ejaculated, he grappled with this new reality, of which I was caught dead smack in the middle. Now, in his mind, he had to reclaim the privileged position of heterosexuality that had been the anchor and foundation of his personality.

In his mind, I was the adversary that stood in the way of his need to rectify the horrible experience that had befallen him. In less clinical terms, homeboy snapped. He was sweating and pacing the floor as he spoke.

"Yo, this was a mistake. You're gonna take yo' ass straight to the press and try to f**k my whole shit up. I can't believe I let a nigga straight f**k me in my ass. What in the hell was I smoking? I can't let you leave until I think this through," he said.

Pause. First, I allow no *trick* to disrespect me. I don't care who the hell they are. Ever. So it was up to me to provide this man with the clarity he desperately needed. Even though I was nervous, I had to appear calm, collected, and in control. These situations did not happen every day in my business, but they did occur, and I already had a process in place to get myself out of there safely. As a call girl, you must think incredibly fast on your feet or perish.

"I know you are experiencing something significant at the moment, but I assure you that my service is confidential. I have a client list of names in my memory that would make your head spin. I do not write pertinent VIP client information down," I said.

Okay, that was a lie. I have always kept a securely encrypted VIP client list for my records. A girl never knows when a circumstance may require the help of a police officer, homicide detective, forensic accountant, police chief, Senator, criminal defense attorney, appellate lawyer, public defender, actor, bad actor, drug dealer, loan shark, convicted felon of some sort, a Mafia made man, a male porn star, restaurateur, CEO, rapper, ballplayer, movie producer, or famous puppeteer...to name a few. Not to mention about 700 garden-variety unfaithful husbands from all races and socioeconomic strata, amassed over 30 years.

As I engaged him in conversation, I nonchalantly made my way toward the hotel room door, monitoring this pressure cooker of a situation without ever losing eye contact with the subject.

"Like I said. I don't trust you," he said.

"Listen, tell yourself whatever you have to for you to be okay. For instance, you were minding your own straight business, and suddenly, through no fault or solicitation of your own, a penis plopped in your mouth and found its way to the crack of your ass. And, of course, at that point, penetration was inevitable. Shit like that happens every day in America," I said.

He glared at me like I was a chalk outline, waiting to happen.

"Okay, maybe that was the wrong imagery to conjure up. Take a second and step back from this situation and digest what you are proposing rationally. You can't just not allow me to leave, right? That's not an option for a few practical reasons. You invited a trans call girl to your hotel room and kept her against her will. A room in a luxury hotel that is registered in your or your agent's name during a scheduled business trip that your itinerary would confirm," I said.

I reached behind and wrapped my right hand around the doorknob as he walked slowly towards me.

"You know what? You are absolutely correct in this situation, and I'm wrong as the day is long. Real talk, I had a good time with your sexy ass, and just couldn't handle it. Like, I was on some vulnerable and scared type shit. But you got my nose open, and I like it. Can I see you again?" he asked.

"Honestly, sweetheart, things like this happen, and all is forgiven. But hell no, I can never see you again, at least not until you get some therapy. No offense, boo, but you're a loose cannon and bad for business. However, if you know any emotionally stable associates in your line of work, who are on the DL like you, give them my number," I replied.

"Naw, baby, I'm not going to refer you to another nigga. I want to deal with you discreetly whenever I can, and I'll deal with what's going on in my head," he said as he attempted to lean in for a kiss.

"I have a pretty good idea how someone like you is going to handle this situation. You're going to profit by repackaging your own sexual insecurities by projecting your superficial hatred of *faggots* and your love for weed and *bitches* through your music and brand messaging. Typical and tired," I said as I averted his kiss and left his suite.

Later that evening, I sat in front of my television in my most comfortable PJs and watched the rapper dazzle onlookers from the red carpet at the Source Awards.

Oh! It was something. He pranced about like a preening peacock. He cocked and crowed before applauding hands and blinking lights. Proud. Unencumbered. His suit of heterosexuality was pressed taut and mitered that night. There wasn't a wrinkle in sight. And before an approving world to see (because he was not careful), his own garment, wore him to a T.

Section 2 (The Cross-Dressing Cokehead)

The buzz from my cell phone broke the peaceful silence that enveloped my modest bedroom. The faint vibration nudged me awake. It was 12:00 AM. I answered the phone, confirmed my rates with the gentleman inquiring about my late-night outcall service, and proceeded to get myself ready.

"Darryl, wake up. I have an outcall to do," I said.

Darryl was my man at the time. He and I were both from Philadelphia, but we had very little else in common. I was pursuing my bachelor's degree in Psychology with a minor in Biology from Florida International University. He had no interest in higher education, and I had no interest in getting high. But for what it was worth, I loved Darryl.

He was supportive, affectionate, and protective. He offered three of the most desired yet rarest qualities found in men who love transgender women. Even if these men possessed these qualities, most of them had little or no interest in displaying these attributes to women like me. I stayed with him, even though, in hindsight, he was as faithful as a condom riddled with bullet holes.

Darryl, like all of the guys I dated at the time, would often travel with me to my outcall appointments or hide in my bedroom closet for an in-call. So if a client broke bad for any reason, my lover was always close by to break their face. Thank God, but I never experienced a physical altercation in my prior profession.

We were in my brand new 2005 White Ford Mustang Convertible by 12:30. "Where are we headed?" he asked.

"Oceania condominiums on 164th and Collins Ave," I replied.

At that time, I lived forty minutes away in Pembroke Pines. The client called me on my cell phone frequently to make sure I was up for the task, literally.

"I'm sorry I keep calling ya, but I just want to make sure that you are totally cool with what I want to go down when you arrive," he said. His speech was fast and erratic. "Wait until you see me. I'm wearing sexy lingerie and cheap hooker boots. Wanna know why I'm wearing cheap hooker boots, Cheyenne? Because I'm a cheap hooker tonight. And you're gonna make me pretty, just like you," he said.

"I'm pulling into guest parking," I said.

"Well then, your sexy ass has been requested to report to Building 1, apartment #2714."

I walked slowly and deliberately to the lobby elevators. It was always a little disconcerting when I had to walk past security to get to my client's condo. In luxury highrises like this, you best believe there are hidden cameras and security posted in every nook and cranny of the property.

"Hello Cheyenne, come on in," he said.

There before me stood a 6'4", 230-pound middle-aged white man, wearing lingerie that was literally bursting at the seams. He had on a dirty blonde, Sally Struthers-type wig that he wore as a hat. It wasn't pulled down securely on his head, the way a wig was designed to be worn.

242

I entered behind him. He clopped around the condo like a silverback mountain gorilla, wearing expensive Anastasia Beverly Hills make-up that sat ashen on his face and high heels four sizes too small. He told me to refer to him as Victoria. He was obviously an aging bodybuilder who was still in pretty decent shape. Victoria's pupils were dilated, and she was sweating like a sow.

He passed me an envelope with approximately $1,500 ducats in it, so I immediately called Darryl to let him I was safe and paid.

"Do you want a bump?" he asked. Big Vicky had a mound of cocaine plopped in the center of a large, thick, beveled glass dining room table. She took a few hits with a rolled-up hundred-dollar bill.

"No, sweetheart. I don't get high. But you can," I said.

She told me that she was on a coke binge that was in its fourth day, and hadn't eaten or slept. I began to watch her very closely for any physical or cognitive signs and symptoms of an impending overdose, while still engaging with her.

When you're doing a lot of cocaine, nothing works. I was hired to dress him like a woman and tell him how pretty he was, period. The first hour went by quickly and without a hitch. Big Vicky was super juiced by this point.

"Can you stay another hour, Cheyenne? I really like you," he commented, between snorts of the white stuff.

"Sure, that will be another donation of $1,500," I said.

"Well, lucky for you, I own about ten Gold's Gyms up and down the east coast. So, I can afford your outrageous rates," he said as he popped a cigarette in his mouth. "But I'm totally out of cash, and I'm too f**ked up to drive to the nearest ATM. I'm gonna give you my Bank of America debit card, my pin number, and the keys to the BMW," coked-out Vicky muttered. She jotted down some numbers on a sticky pad and grabbed her car keys out of the mahogany curio cabinet that stood in the corner of the room.

"Uh! Are you sure you want to give me your banking information? You don't even know me," I asked.

"Don't let the hair, dress, and make-up fool ya. I'm an excellent judge of character. I'm a big Italian guy from the Bronx. I know that you're a smart, no-nonsense,

and all business kinda girl. Am I wrong?"
she said.

"You know what? This sounds strange. I
mean, you could report your card and car
stolen and put my black ass in jail," I
responded.

"And oh, I forgot paranoid. Call the
cops! Call the cops! Are you crazy? I got
enough cocaine hidden in my apartment that
could get the entire Miami Beach Police
department as high as hell. And most of
those pricks buy from me, by the way," she
said.

I grabbed everything I needed except
the car keys. On the elevator down to the
lobby, I explained the entire situation to
Darryl. He was waiting in the passenger
seat in front of the Oceania. The Bank
of America was only a few blocks south on
Collins Ave. There we were, driving down
the avenue in Sunny Isles in the middle
of the night, with a strange white man's
bank card and PIN. That entire scene gave
me the willies. And if my memory serves
me correctly, I might have been driving on
a suspended license, at that. Talk about
choices.

I parked discreetly in a space just a
few feet away from the bank's ATM. I looked

around to make sure no one had pulled into the lot behind us. The shopping center where the Bank of America was at was totally vacant at 3 a.m. I took a deep breath, inserted the card, and punched in the six-digit password on the back of the sticky note.

"Oh my God," I screamed.

"Shh! What the hell you screaming for, boo? Is you alright?" Darryl said.

"Darryl, come here quick," I gasped, frantically waving at the car.

Darryl tentatively approached the ATM and stood next to me.

"Get the f**k outta here," he yelled.

"Shh," I whispered.

Well, there it was in black and white (no pun intended). Big Vicky had big bucks. There was an open savings account with more than $3 million and a checking account totaling over $750,000. Darryl and I both stood there glaring at the ATM screen with our mouths open, dumbfounded. I had never seen that much money in a bank account, or in any other form, in my life.

"Wow! Somebody needs to rob that muthaf***a," he said.

"Baby, are you just that high, or just that stupid?"

" I'm just sayin'. I know you're not a thief, and that's one of the many qualities about you that I love. But do you know how many trans girls I know in Philly that would set that fool up and rob him? Know how many I know? All of them. Every last one. All day. Without question," Darryl said.

"Well, what I'm gonna do is withdraw exactly what he and I agreed on, and not a dollar more. I am not playing with this crazy white man and his money," I said.

I took out enough for two more sessions and returned to the apartment. By the time I returned, Big Vicky was drenched in sweat and barely coherent. I thought to myself, *How much cocaine could he have snorted? I was only gone twenty minutes.*

I placed the bank card and sticky note in the palm of his hand and grabbed a 2-liter bottle of water from the refrigerator. "Here, Mrs. Vicky girl, drink some of this," I said.

Big Vicky grabbed the bottle of water and made her way into the living room when I heard a loud crash. It was the sound of glass breaking with a huge thud.

I ran into the living room from the kitchen. Big Vicky had fallen through the center of the oversized beveled glass table, where she lay motionless.

I hoisted my dress up to my thighs, kicked off my heels, and kneeled beside his head. His pupils were fixed and dilated. And I was unable to feel a pulse — anywhere. This man did not have an apical, radial, popliteal, or carotid pulse. I desperately checked them all, just in case one of them was on vacation. Basically, this man had dropped dead of an overdose. My pulse, on the other hand, was pounding out of my chest.

Now, this situation would qualify as one of those forks in the road, moments when a whore has a sidebar with herself, to reevaluate her life choices, occupation, and aspirations. But there was no time. I just did not have the luxury of feeling sorry for myself…or the dead man on the floor wearing lingerie. I had to shove that money-grubbing whore, Cheyenne, to the back of my mind and summon Jasmine, the telemetry nurse, to the front.

I checked the body to make sure there weren't any problematic lacerations from the glass. I placed him flat on his back and ran down the basic CPR checklist in my head.

First, call 911. Well, I wasn't doing
that. That was entirely out of the question,
at least until I performed three unsuccess-
ful rounds of CPR. I was a black transgen-
der call-girl entertaining a wealthy white
cross-dressing businessman and/or whole-
sale drug dealer in Sunny Isles, and had
just made a late-night withdrawal from his
bank account.

Second, I opened his mouth to make sure
he had a clear airway. Third, I checked for
pulse and breathing. He had neither. Fourth,
I did something that I wouldn't recommend
doing. However, these were desperate times.
I delivered two rescue breaths by pinch-
ing his nose, cupping my free hand to form
a loose hole with my fingers, and blowing
steadily and deeply. Fifth, I unhooked the
corset he had on, straddled his chest, and
performed 30 chest compressions, two fin-
gers width apart from the xiphoid process.

I moved fast and methodically during
all of this. I was working as a per diem
telemetry nurse at the time. I knew the
longer he was without oxygen, the more
tissue damage there would be if I were to
eventually get a pulse.

After the first round of CPR, I still
couldn't feel a pulse and started the

second round. At that point, I was incredibly nervous, and my brain was operating a mile a minute. I was thinking like a nurse and Sherlock Holmes at the same time.

I thought about the optics of the situation in the event I had to call the police. Could I adequately explain the circumstances surrounding the sudden collapse of my client? No, I couldn't. I was halfway through the second round of CPR when I did something peculiar.

I delivered six consecutive rescue breaths and 30 subsequent chest compressions. I then ran into his bedroom to look for his regular clothes. I revisited the most critical step in the CPR series — call 911. In between chest compressions and rescue breaths, I undressed and redressed my client in male clothes. After the fourth round of CPR, I felt a slight pulse. He was alive, and there was no time to lose. I delivered two more rescue breaths and turned him on his side. His breathing improved, and the color came back into his ashen face.

While he was recuperating on the floor, now dressed as a man, I proceeded to wipe my fingerprints off of every object in the apartment I thought I might have touched.

I wiped down the countertops, all of the doorknobs in and out of the apartment, and especially that damn Bank of America debit card. By the time I finished doing all of that, he was sitting on the floor in smudged make-up and jogging pants.

"Did I stop breathing again?" he asked.

"Uh, yeah, you stopped breathing. I couldn't find a pulse, so I started performing CPR on you."

"Oh wow, really? The last girl I saw didn't do that. When I came to, she was gone," he said.

"I'm a nurse. Wait. Again? The last girl? This has happened before?"

"Oh yeah, when I get really f***ed up. I have a preexisting medical condition. So, when I go on my coke binges, I have stopped breathing for up to three and a half minutes. My heart rate will bottom down to around 20 beats a minute," he said as he attempted to scoop up some of the cocaine residue from the broken glass table.

"No, this time, you had no pulse. You f***in' cokehead asshole. Listen to me very carefully before you take another f***in' hit of anything. You overgrown drag queen drug addict. You will erase all of the text messages between you and me regarding my escort service immediately. You will then send me a text message thanking me for my assistance in helping you construct your modified cross-training regimen for medically vulnerable populations at your gym. The payment for the aforementioned service will be the exact amount that was withdrawn from your account earlier," I said.

I took his cell phone and called myself. Keep me on the line until I reach Pembroke Pines.

"Clever girl. A regular black Nancy Drew," he said.

"Nancy Drew this, dickwad. If you really want to kill yourself, Bronx boy, don't be a pussy about it. Get some guts. And give yourself a hot shot of Potassium chloride, boo-boo," I said as I exited the apartment.

"Is that the professional opinion of the nurse or the prostitute, sweetheart?" he yelled as the door closed behind me.

Section 3 (Trade Who Didn't Know He Was Trade)

In this section, I feel the need to clarify gay and trans slang for my unfamiliar readers. Men who fall into the category of trade are not gay-identified but engage in intimate acts with individuals of the same sex. This term was initially ascribed to the young hyper-masculine male of minority race who fitted a particular thug stereotype and who "traded" sex for money with gay men. Over the years, the term trade has come to identify closeted men of any race or ethnicity who live as heterosexuals, but engage in casual and sometimes anonymous sex with gay men for money and/or fun.

Transgender women often regard trans-attracted men who are not open about their sexual orientation as trade. The term was always used in a flippant, pejorative manner. Why? I can only communicate my own thoughts on the matter. Trade and DL men are arguably cut from the same cloth. They indulge in what I describe as double-dipping.

Historically, these individuals siphon sexual, emotional, and psychological fulfillment from one group while clinging to the other group's privilege. Although I am aware of the reason for this behavior and the social ramifications surrounding planting one's flag in the less empowered minority group's soil, I am not a fan of such foolishness. As a transgender woman, this concept has often been the bane of my existence. It contributes to my less supportive view of those caught in this matrix. So in saying that, the idea of disclosing one's gender identity also requires the same level of scrutiny and introspection.

I met Mike at the Bethlehem public library when I was twenty years old. That would make it around 1992. It was a beautiful summer day. I had already begun taking hormones and started to develop breasts. I never grew facial hair, just peach fuzz, really. I was short, thin, bow-legged with medium chestnut-colored eyes.

I remember having a signature look back then: I wore long brown micro-braids, tight short shorts, and fitted blouses that framed my foam falsies, enhancing my budding bosoms. And in the winter, I would change up that ensemble by adding a coat. So, I had a pretty cute thing going on – for a newbie.

Before information flowed effortlessly with the stroke of a finger, when that digital superhighway was nothing more than a one-lane road that ended in a cul-de-sac, the Bethlehem Public Library stood as a beacon of knowledge and a centralized hub for social gatherings and activities of all kinds. Of course, I was there not to read but to cruise.

This is where another gay slang tutorial may be in order. Cruising, to put it politely, was fleeting sex between men or transgender women (for the purpose of this book), usually anonymously and often in semi-public indoor or outdoor spaces. I personally was there to flirt and mingle with guys, as I was all dolled up, but the company I kept was undoubtedly there to cruise.

The first time I ever laid eyes on Mike, he was jogging down North New Street to the library. I wasn't very attracted to white men in my youth, but something about him physically did it for me. Mike had a rugged look and demeanor that I found attractive. Although classically Caucasian, his blond hair and incredible blue eyes were placed on a man who stood 6'4" with a muscular build and spoke and acted like he was born and bred in somebody's projects. And that contrast was so hot. He had an affinity for Black and Spanish women, which made total sense.

He asked me out on a date, and I accepted. When trans women are typically approached by men, we have a tendency to search their face and body language to determine whether they have discovered our "feminine uniqueness" at any point during the conversation.

Mike did not. It was a lovely, breezy summer afternoon, so we decided to take a pleasant stroll down to Monocacy Creek. Sad to say, given my character in those early days, I wound up performing oral sex on this man while he stood against a tree, in broad daylight. I knew him all of an hour, tops. Talk about choices on both of our ends. And my eagerness to put my mouth on him should have been a big blaring sign that something was amiss. It is not common for attractive cisgendered (biological) females to give blow jobs, even to handsome strangers, without the inhibition-lowering effects of drugs or alcohol, minus the exchange of money.

He didn't pick up the fact that my sexual openness was a classic display of transgender behavior. Behavior I am proud to say I later grew out of.

What I came to like most about Mike was that he was very generous and honest.

"Jasmine, I realize that this is our first date, but I want to be totally straight with you," Mike said.

I looked him in the eyes with bated breath as my Diana Ross-style hair weave fluttered past my shoulders. Our dinner table at the Chinese restaurant was directly underneath a softly humming air conditioner that tossed my hair gently.

"You can tell me anything, Mike. I'm a very understanding girl," I said.

"Well, I'm in recovery, first of all. And I have been drug-free for several years. I tell any woman that I date my story because I don't want to mislead anybody. My sobriety and my two little girls mean everything to me. And if a woman wants to be a part of my life, she has to accept me for who I am. Understand that staying clean is a choice. I choose each day whether or not I will let the stresses or pressure of the day convince me to take a crack pipe to the head. I make fifty thousand a year, and I am happier than I have ever been. All I need is a beautiful woman like you by my side," he said.

"Wow! Thank you for trusting me with your story, Mike," I replied.

"Anything you wanna tell me or get out in the open. Like a crazy ex or current boyfriend I may have to beat down?" he asked with a smirk as he licked his lips. Homeboy had a lip-licking L.L. Cool J kinda vibe happening. I felt a tugging in my heart, and I was compelled to reveal my deepest truth.

"Mike, I too have something to tell you about myself that may or may not be obvious. But I need to tell you and pray that you accept me for who I am," I said nervously.

"I really dig you J, you can tell me anything. I'm really falling for you, baby," he said calmly. "What is it."

"I know you think I'm this beautiful girl, but I'm a beautiful girl with a secret," I said.

"What is it, baby?" he repeated.

"Mike, sweetheart. I am so sorry to tell you, but my hair isn't real. I wear something called hair weaves. As a matter of fact, I'm sporting the Diana Ross, the missing Mahogany years limited edition, in human hair, 1B."

"Is that it?"

"Not quite. I wear fake acrylic nails too," I said as I wiggled my nails in his face.

We bared our souls to one another over moo shu pork, beef and broccoli, and spare rib tips. Well, at least he did.

We began a whirlwind romance. We dated heavily for about three months. Mike was exceptionally kind, patient, and sensitive to my needs as a woman. So I didn't want a little insignificant fact relating to my gender to hinder our happiness. Right? Wrong!

Like I communicated in Chapter two, I have lived in the Lehigh Valley since I was eight years old. I don't know what made me think that I could openly date a man, with me dressed as a woman, in the same town I grew up in. This is the kind of dumb bullshit we spoon-feed ourselves so we can rest more comfortably when the sun goes down.

I knew I was transgender, even if he did not at the time. I allowed him to parade me around town, holding my hand, because it made me feel normal and loved. And parenthetically speaking, his identity as a man, his reputation, the opinion of his children and his sobriety were inconsequential and took a back seat to my inflated ego and gender dysphoria. One day several months after we had been dating, someone pulled Mike aside, whispered something in his ear, and in a nutshell, this was the outcome.

He was devastated. He had taken me to meet his mother, sponsor, and a host of his friends. He expressed his love for me to them as often as anyone would let him. Initially, like some men, he tried to convince himself that the fact that I was born male, and still, at that point, had a penis, wasn't a barrier that love couldn't overcome. He clung to images of me that reinforced my femininity, like how I made him feel sexually. Still, those feelings left him confused and conflicted about his own sexual orientation. That didn't work. We couldn't work.

We broke up, and because we genuinely cared about each other, we tried our hand at being friends. But the betrayal of me not disclosing my gender to him much earlier in our relationship so he could make an informed decision "played on the tracks of his mind, like an old scratched vinyl record."

After two weeks of him discovering I was transgender, we never spoke again...for fifteen years.

I kept my ears to the streets after that and discovered Mike had relapsed and lost his job due to depression and crack cocaine addiction. I subsequently relocated to Miami, where I transformed myself into the sultry, eye-popping Jasmine many came to love – and pay for.

Fifteen years later, in 2005, I got a friendship request from a guy with the same name as his. I accepted the request. I needed to apologize and hear that he was all right after all these years. We exchanged numbers, and this was the gist of that much-anticipated conversation.

"Hello, Mike," I said.

"Hello, Jasmine. How have you been?" he asked.

"This is so surreal that I'm talking to you right now. There are some things I need to say before we get sidetracked by all of this small talk," I said.

"Okay. You first, then me," he said.

"Mike, I have wanted to apologize for the past fifteen years. I am so sorry for the hurt I have caused you. I can't imagine what meeting me cost you. You were so good to me, and I got caught up in a lot of fear of losing that feeling of safety and security you gave me. I'm older, but more importantly, I've gotten some much-needed therapy. Trans women are frequently relegated to society's fringes and left to fend for themselves in a cruel, dark world, merely because people don't understand their gender dysphoria. That kind of loneliness and rejection contribute to some very questionable behavior. That realization doesn't make me any less exempt from living a more authentic life. If anything, it makes me more culpable. In saying this, I chose to embark on this life's journey in a woman's body. I learned that it was also my responsibility to disclose my gender identity to a potential partner before becoming intimate. Everyone has the right to choose who they want to be intimate with. It was wrong for me to project my identity onto you, unsuspectedly. I heard you had a tough time after was broke up," I said.

"Wow! You just look and sound so different. You became the woman that you always thought you should have been. And I accept that lengthy-ass apology. Damn, Jasmine. You were talking as though you were accepting an Academy Award or something. But seriously, yes, I did have a rough time. When I saw you, I thought you had a unique look that I was attracted to. And just like an addict, I wanted what I wanted. In hindsight, were there any signs? Of course. I really liked what we had going on, and then you became another kind of drug to me. We had a lot of oral and anal sex that I had never experienced before. I became addicted to you and how you made me feel like a man. But when other people told me who you were, it was like the fantasy I had created was exposed. And when my Jasmine high was not available, I resorted back to my original drug of choice. I did blame you for my relapse. I learned at my meetings that getting high is always a choice for the addict, regardless of life's stressors or pressures. I am now married with 2 more kids and couldn't be happier. And it looks like you found happiness as well," Mike said.

We laughed, reminisced, and caught each other up on the last fifteen years of our lives. We finally had the closure both of us needed. After that conversation, Mike de-friended me, and we never spoke again.

Chapter 6:   But God

Flawed Human Nature

We tread on the past lives of
others.

Unencumbered. Dogmatic and
entitled.

Superimposing our will onto
theirs, As if we've

already bought the rights to
tomorrow.
Striding as though it is
not HE, but we, who make
ourselves.

Step by step, we roam the
earth, fooling ourselves into
believing-

our lives are the only lives
worths living,

in the annals of all breaths
taken.

We think inept thoughts,
vascillating between cognitive
voids

And psychological tsunamis.

We are irretrievably flawed,
and our cantankerous
nature- contagious.

We think with small minds but
play with big guns.

We are a scary and present
danger to our whole being.

Until ushered into the cold
ground. And we, too, are
trotted over by the brethren.

August 18th, 2016

J.C. Ford

Section 1 (The Fifth Encounter: The Great Melting)

In Acts 9 in the Bible, Saul had his converting encounter with the Lord on a dusty road traveling from Jerusalem to Damascus over 2,000 years ago. I met HIM in a little modest baptist church situated on the corner of Goepp and New Street in Bethlehem when I was 13 years old. And that great introduction was my third encounter with God. That precious life-disruptive blessing has kept me ever since, despite and in conflict with my sexuality.

I fell in love with God like a lovesick schoolgirl in my late thirties. Although I became saved as a teenager, life's circumstances pulled me away from my faith further than I ever imagined.

It's hard to pray when you're a prostitute. When you have laid down with so many men, that time, faces and details are a blur—a crippling collage of memories too vivid to forget and too painful to recall. Where spiritually and carnally, my "soured insides reeked of spoiled cabbage, salve, and ointment" all because "my supple flesh ripe for the right price, now wept with decay."

The conversations with my Father God always left me in a pool of tears as I lay prostrate beside my bed. The shame and guilt were psychologically paralyzing at times. Still, faith drove me to my knees because deliverance was coming. Yet, I still believed HIM for the great melting that would justify and sanctify me. The immutable word of God dictated it would. All I had were HIS promises.

And lo, they come to pass without provocation and without any warning.

Blessings just fell from the sky like rainbow-colored gumdrops one day, and I was the kid on the playground with the biggest sweet tooth.

I picked up Raquel for church like I had been doing almost every Sunday since we had met in 2011. It was in December 2015. I had been a dedicated member of New Birth Baptist Church for as long as I've known the clan.

It had been about 7 years since I had that experience on the 5th floor of the Red Roof Inn in Washington, D.C., that drove me back into the sanctuary, straight into the arms of Jesus Christ. What I saw and heard within the four walls of that room further solidified my belief in Heaven and

Hell. Although my life was spared on that hot afternoon in that dingy hotel room, my spirit was still broken. And I was expecting a miracle every time I entered the sanctuary.

I couldn't accurately articulate what my soul needed to make it whole again. All I knew was that the darkness had "sprouted big, brazen roots that wormed down deep, and anchored my soul in soured oil."

During praise and worship, the choir began to sing the song, 'Something Happens'(When you call Him: Jesus, Jesus, Jesus). I started to worship in the spirit in that crowded sanctuary like I was an audience of one. Crying out to HIM in confusion, desperation, and despair. Truly praising him for who HE was and not what HE could do for me. I praised in total admiration until tears streamed down my face, staining my blouse with make-up. And then, I felt the presence of the Holy Spirit-heavy in the atmosphere. The initial outpouring crashed against me like a tidal wave in the fifth row of the pews. With the air thick with his glory and power, I humbled myself. I "became as low as a slug," and my soul sang psalms of contrition."

Before I could steady myself, the second wave made me buckle to my knees. I was disoriented. I felt HIM everywhere. The sensation and emotion of unfathomable love HE had for me felt like it permeated every fiber of my being. Every individual cell in my body somehow recognized that its creator had manifested, and for a particular reason.

My purse that was resting on the pew fell to the ground. Money that was folded in a tight wad, earned from the night before, rolled onto the green carpet. My best friend Raquel came to my aid and tried to keep me from hitting the floor. My body went limp.

The third wave enveloped me. And I heard very distinctly, " It's going to be alright," echoing on a whisper of wind. Those words, as simple as they were, broke me down so my soul could open up. And it did. I was experiencing my great melting.

Little Jof was the first to emerge, less afraid of the ugly that had encapsulated him for so long. Fortified with the gift of forgiveness, he began to run, leap and catapult off the ball of his feet. Still, not a boy. Still, not a girl. And felt less like an alien, visiting your world.

James wept.

The one who believed that peace and happiness could be found on the receiving end of a surgeon's scalpel became all body and no substance.

Believing that she embodied the ugliness of unworthiness, simply found worth in becoming someone else. Clutched those lies tightly to her bare breast and breathed on them. While never asking God what HE thought about her.

Consequently, Jasmine foolishly and tediously tended to the chaff in her life while her wheat withered away. But, the restorer was in the building that morning. The God that "chose things the world considers foolish in order to shame those who think they are wise. And HE chose things that are powerless to shame those who are powerful."

The Holy Spirit held Cheyenne the whore the longest because her scars were the deepest and freshest. We all wept in the sanctuary that morning during that great melting. The Lord will always require you to participate in your healing or deliverance. HE left some work for me to do on my own, but I felt like I was created for a purpose that extended beyond my minuscule comprehension for the first time in my life. I was finally determined to capture my divinely ordained purpose-driven life.

But wait, there are serpents in the sanctuary...

Section 2 (Serpents in the Sanctuary)

Believe it or not, but my exodus out of the hottest party town in the country, to Fredericksburg, Virginia, had its genesis in church. During the spring of 2016, I attended a woman's conference at the church I was a member. If my memory serves me correctly, I believe Bishop McCullough, a notable pastor was one of the speakers during the week-long event. I went by myself, and there was a mighty move of God during the service as she preached passionately about the posture of women of faith. In keeping with the spirit of forgiveness that was the biblical theme that evening, the Bishop asked something bold of the female churchgoers. She instructed individuals in the pews to seek out another woman that she may have wronged in some form or another, but the devil had kept them from making amends. The Holy

Spirit had a heavy presence in the sanctuary, as people were moved in their hearts to repair relationships through contrition with one another.

I hadn't wronged anyone in the church, to my knowledge. So I continued to stand in place in silent prayer, praise, and support as participants scurried around the large sanctuary, hugging and crying. It was beautiful to see a room full of women from every walk of life attempting to heal old wounds in real-time. I felt blessed and privileged to be a witness to such an event.

I accepted and gave hugs as they were offered. So it was not a surprise to me when a woman I barely recognized walked in my direction, weaving in and out of the pews, as she made her way to me. I remember that her eyes were blood-sight, puffy, and filled with water. Her lower lip trembled as she got closer.

"Hello, Jasmine. Do you remember who I am," the lady said.

"Yes, of course, I believe we went to nursing school together. But you were a class ahead of me. So, how are you," I responded.

I most certainly did remember her. She would give me dirty looks every time she would encounter me fifteen years earlier. She would tell other student nurses that I was really a "man" and laugh. She was Haitian, so I would often catch her speaking French and pointing menacingly in my direction. I experienced my share of bullying while attempting to get my education.

"I am so sorry, Jasmine, but I have wronged you in the worst way, and I needed you to know that. I also hope you can find it in your heart to forgive me," she confessed, as more tears rolled down her face.

I moved a little closer to her to appear more open and engaging. I was ready and willing to receive a heartfelt apology for her cruelty to me when we were in our early and mid-twenties matriculating through nursing school. But I was absolutely not ready for what would precede out of the mouth of that teary-eyed viper.

"I'm the reason that you haven't been able to get a job with some of the medical facilities in the area. I am now the Dean of Nursing, and she stated the facility where she worked. You came into my facility for an interview and did very well,

I heard. When I saw you, I immediately remembered you from school. Not only did I not hire you at my facility, but I also faxed your resume to other DON's at other local medical facilities. I stated that you were a man dressed like a woman seeking a nursing job. I also said that I had it on good authority that your clinical skills and mental health were in question. Someone like you would be a professional liability. I knowingly misrepresented your character as a nurse simply because you are trans. That was wrong, and if there is anything I can do to assist you in finding employment, Jasmine, I am ready to do that for you. Can you forgive me?" she said.

The palms of my hands became clammy. There was a sudden tightness in my chest. I felt light-headed, as though I might lose my balance and faint at any moment. I stumbled backward a few steps in utter shock and disbelief. I had to grab onto the back of a pew to restore my balance.

Her confession was so incredibly unsettling. I had been actively looking for employment for the past 2 years. I couldn't figure out for the life of me why I either wasn't landing any preliminary interviews or wasn't being considered for a job. I brushed up on both my clinical skills and my interviewing techniques; to no avail. I wanted to get back into nursing and went to great lengths to obtain employment.

My inability to find a job literally almost drove me insane. I edited my resume 3 times. By the 4th edit, I embellished my clinical knowledge and experience so badly in desperation, it was embarrassing. I yoyoed between wearing make-up and going fresh-faced to the few interviews I landed, to wearing a polyester 2 piece suit or scrubs. One has to be woefully desperate, fashionably inept, or crazy as hell to put on a Hilary Clinton type polyester two-piecer, in Miami and think it's cute.

By this time, I was approaching my mid-forties, and the escort business had contorted my mind, body, and spirit. I wanted out but didn't know how to escape. All of my efforts over the last couple of years hadn't materialized into any significant progress. And a huge chunk of that reason was standing right in front of me in the middle of a Gospel Women's Conference, focusing on Solidarity and Sisterhood. The irony of the situation was so palpable, you could slice it with a knife.

But the conversation did not end there. I hadn't responded yet.

"Wait! Let me get this straight. You mean to tell me that you're the reason why I couldn't get a nursing job between Miami and West Palm Beach over the last few years.? Like, How is that possible? All this time, I thought something was wrong with me. You don't understand, I felt that I might have harmed a patient and wasn't aware of it, but others were. A million different scenarios fluttered my mind on what could be the issue. And you mean to tell me that one transphobic pseudo-Christian in the right position of power is all it took? "You fork-tongued serpent, I rebuke you in the name of Jesus Christ. And, although I will forgive you because forgiveness is Godly, but it damn sure won't be today," I said.

I left the sanctuary that evening, first of all, relieved that I wasn't losing my mind surrounding my employment situation. But with a renewed dedication to correct the course that my life was on. Come hell or high water, as God is my secret judge, I made a promise to myself that I was not going to die on the streets of Miami, a prostitute. I was too intelligent, too talented, and too blessed for such a sad, unremarkable narrative to be my legacy on this earth. With tears streaming down my face, I claimed that affirmation with everything inside of me, in the mighty name of Jesus Christ.

Darkest Before Dawn

My colored is crude.
Seared on by blood,
Sweat and tears.
A million lashes and
400 years.
Oh yes indeed,
My colored is costly,
But my faith is free.
You see,
Balanced   against the
Opposition of my blackness,
The relative condition
Of my freedom,
Is ongoing conjecture,
I have with my maker.
Oh yes I concede.
My colored is crushing,
But my faith freed me.

J.C. Ford

Section 3 (Fredericksburg, Virginia: Welcome to FAHASS)

The very next day, I woke up early, opened my laptop to indeed.com, and began a new job search. I spoke to the Lord most of the night and concluded that I had to take ownership of the part I played in my own professional demise. After all, I advertised my "provider services" throughout South Florida for over 20 years in publications such as the Miami Herald, New Times, Sexaction Magazine, Taboo Magazine, and internationally in Eros guide. Even though I operated under an alias, I utilized actual photos of myself. In doing so, established credibility in a business where catfishing was the norm than the outlier. However, this helped build a solid reputation in high-end escort work, making it increasingly difficult for me as a nurse. So with this realization brewing in the back of my brain, I expanded my search beyond South Florida and job title boundaries. If I were going to start fresh, I would do so in an unprecedentedly transparent way. I uploaded a resume and cover letter that disclosed that I was a transgender nurse of color with a great deal of experience looking for a fresh start.

I nervously pressed the send button and waited with bated breath.

To my surprise and delight, things moved incredibly fast. Interest in my skills and background came pouring in from around the country. Have I missed something? Since when did medical facilities, agencies, and companies actively recruit transgender individuals? Well, I certainly wasn't going to look a gift horse in the mouth or over-analyze myself right out of an opportunity. I immediately took an interest in four emails from organizations and clinics across the country that provided medical and supportive services to individuals diagnosed with HIV. Although I was a nurse, I had little practical experience with this patient population. Most of my clinical experience was on a cardiac step-down unit. When I did come in contact with patients with HIV, their admission diagnosis was cardiac-related.

The thought of providing assistance to individuals living with the chronic disorder of HIV tugged at my heartstrings. It filled my spirit once again with an overwhelming sense of gratitude and purpose. I knew that familiar feeling. The Holy Spirit was telling me to go. He was etching my earthly assignment on the surface of my heart in the spirit. Not just to change my life, but hopefully to impact others.

I refamiliarized myself with the human immunodeficiency virus. I researched viral morphology, its transmission, to the advancement in pharmacokinetics. I wasn't going to be rejected for lack of knowledge, that was for damn sure.

I set up 4 in-person interviews with Mazzoni Center in Philadelphia, Fredericksburg Area HIV/AIDS Support Services in Fredericksburg, Virginia, Howard Brown Health in Chicago, Illinois, and an HIV/ Drug Rehabilitation Center in Frederick, Maryland.

After flying across the country, in some instances twice, for a second interview, I was offered a position at Fredericksburg Area HIV/AIDS Support Services (FAHASS) and accepted.

I honestly had a rough start at FAHASS despite how eager I was to leave the escort profession alone. Although the Lord had healed me from many of the traumas and suicidal ideation I had experienced during the great melting, He left work for me to accomplish on my own. The work I had to do on my own made me challenge a lifestyle I had become intimately acquainted with. On some subconscious level, I was reticent to say goodbye despite the harm it caused and the deliverance I received.

Just like Neil Gaiman warns in his book The Graveyard, "Wherever you go, you take yourself with you," but in my case, this assertion didn't entirely ring true. I had a fair starting salary of $46,000 a year. Thus, by all accounts and considering my circumstances, the organization provided me a tremendous financial and professional introduction back into the workforce.

By 2017, I had become completely frustrated with my living conditions in Fredericksburg, and I was contemplating returning to Miami, where I had more access to resources. Let me explain. Although I absolutely loved working with the client population in which we served at FAHASS, I hadn't precisely settled myself into the suburban lifestyle. You see, in South Florida, I lived a posh lifestyle because I had sex with wealthy, well-connected men. I had jacked up credit, but I always lived in beautiful condos throughout Dade and Broward County. How? Men.

I found myself unable to find an apartment to rent even though I was gainfully employed due to my terrible credit history. So, I was forced to live in hotels to the tune of $3,000 a month. Not including food, gas, or my car note.

I soon called on my oldest profession without the experience, sex appeal, intuition, quick wit, and overt sexuality of Cheyenne. Instead, I was delivered of my alter-ego, or she of me, during the great melting. I haven't been able to conjure her up since. So, I was on my own. And that was not good because Jasmine was terrible at it. You can't turn a trick with a lot of nervous stuttering and stammering going on.

As a result of my sudden inexperience at a job I had been doing literally for over 30 years, I was arrested. I was cuffed not for prostitution but for a misdemeanor charge called living and dwelling in a bawdy place. Basically, an accusation states that one is keeping, residing in, or visiting a place for immoral purposes. I was devastated!

I was in jail for 2 days, but I carried on as though I was facing a life sentence. I was trying the pray the grey sky blue. When I say, I prayed like I was crazy. I prayed until I was horse, and sweat poured from my brow. I rebuked the devil and sent him crashing down to the pit of hell a few times during my stay. He was every liar in the book.

I must have been praying in repetition and stereo because a voice shouted out during one of my prayer breaks, " Oh listen, the tranny whore knows the Lord," an inmate said.

"That's right! Call me Mary Magdalene, you dirty dick convict," I responded.

And moments later, it happened—the selfless gesture that changed the trajectory of my life professionally, psychologically, and spiritually.

A day and a half earlier, when I was instructed to make my phone call, the only number I knew by heart was my work number. So, I swallowed my pride, or what was left of it, and placed a direct call to my employer. At the time, the Care Services Program Manager, named Joseph, drove one hundred miles round trip twice to see his employee in jail. Joseph traveled from Fredericksburg to Richmond to visit me after working a full eight-hour day and back home. And the following day, he returned late at night to bail me out of jail and stayed until I was released well after 1:00

a.m. in the morning. God had answered my prayers once again.

The amount of love, support, and compassion the entire agency showed towards me during my worst time was astounding. Joseph permitted me to retain my position as Medical Case Manager, disregarding the resignation letter I had given him weeks earlier. I am so thankful that I didn't experience any backlash or been the subject of office gossip. Nor did I ever experience any micro-aggression from my peers due to my arrest ,or the nature of the charges.

I had experienced the fourth wave of the Great Melting at Fredericksburg Area HIV/AIDS Support Services. The God-ordained human capacity to love, forgive and grow. This wave hit me just as hard as the first three because I wasn't prepared to receive such blessings through mankind by Christ.

It healed something in me that had been broken for many years- my sense of identity and belonging.

There was light, where there was once darkness and despair. That's what happens when you find your purpose.

Armed with a renewed sense of self, I took off. I began to take the lead on projects and tasks. In addition, I actively pursued knowledge surrounding HIV care services and Ryan White Funding outside the purview of my current job position.

In May 2018, I was sworn in as a Commissioner on the Washington, DC Regional Planning Commission on Health and HIV. A new regional planning body for HIV prevention and care services in the federally defined Washington, DC Eligible Metropolitan Area. My new life was beginning to take shape as my career took flight.

In the summer of 2020, I was promoted to Programs Manager of the largest department in the organization. Good Ol' Joseph, my boss, mentor, and friend, accepted the position as Executive Director of the agency a few years prior.

I marvel at what God can do with the foolish things. I was extricated out of the muck and mire of a destructive life, cleansed, and placed on a new journey with his WORD "as a lamp unto my feet and a light unto my path." And now I can finally declare with surety, that I know who I am.

Depending on who you ask, I may be described as a beautiful lie, due to my gender identity. But watch in angst, as this beautiful lie, through the power and grace of God, learned how to fly.

I Know Who I Am

Lacking power of perfusion,
Your negative assessment
Won't quicken me to draw
An empty breath.
You smote down beast of the deep.
I resign unto you nothing.
Not err shred of dignity,
Nor morsel of self-respect.
But, instead, watch in angst as
I stand forever firm footed
On the precipice of my tomorrow.
A nudging wind at my back-
Flicking me forward.
The golden lights of heaven
warming my face
Sanctioning my soul,
Fully persuaded that I am
remarkably created.

J.C. Ford

Chapter 7: In Reflection

I wrote this book because, like many of us, the CoronaVirus (COVID-19) had robbed me of the natural order of my life. And I began to drown in my own sense of helplessness as I helplessly watched the death toll mount over the months. So, in a fit of defiant spiritual retaliation, I challenged myself to do what was within my power to make better in a world crippled by a virus - and I started with me.

I knew I needed to write a book that was a direct antithesis to the energy that had been opportunistically feeding off of the love, peace and joy so many people exude on a daily basis, throughout the world. And if transgender people are anything, we are brave, and pride ourselves on facing insurmountable challenges head on, particularly when the odds are against us. I took up that mantle like I had so many times before, and *Flight of the Beautiful Lie* is the result. People needed to hear a different narrative about the trans experience that didn't end in tragedy, but could be utilized as a beautiful beacon of hope, light and love for all the world to see. As you have read, I am most certainly a flawed human being, but in the prophetic words of Miss Celie, "I'm here. Thank God I'm here."

Nothing is more egoistic and inaccurate, when individuals pretend that God had absolutely nothing to do with the success and peace they are blessed to be experiencing. And it was to that end, why I had to approach this manuscript with unrelenting honesty and candor. The blessings of others depended upon it.

I wrote at times, in the wee hours of the morning, with tears streaming down my face, all because God thought I was worthy. So I wrote at the expense of myself and what harm the information within the pages of this book could do in the wrong hands. Still, I chose to believe God.

And for those of you who don't know the saving and redemptive love of Jesus Christ, give HIM a try. The Great Melting isn't just a singular experience, for a single individual. The Great Melting is available to all who believe in HIM for your healing mind, body and spirit.

I look forward to many of you opening the pages of my next book. The prequel to The Great Melting, called *The Great Introduction*.....

Summer's Day

Sun rays splash against moist brown skin,
Painting me a darker hue.
Bare feet meet prickly shards of grass.
Cool morning dew trickle between my toes.
I smile wide, as a swirl of wind
tickles my nose.
Stalks of bundled wool crown my head-
Course and nappy.
Before a gigglin' God,
I stand bow legged
Black, blessed and happy.
On this summer's day.

J.C. Ford

The End... Of volume one that is.

Photo Gallery

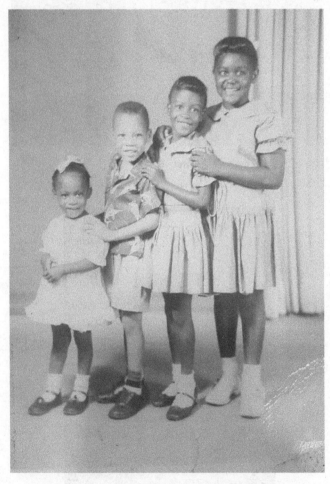

pick of 4 siblings in order of birth
The smallest:
Carla, William (Sunny), Tina, Alease Ford

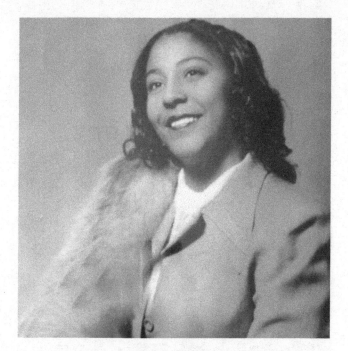

Aunt Mary

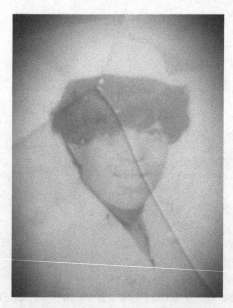

Pic of mother Carla Ford high
school graduation photo

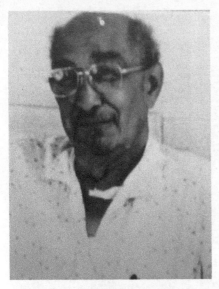

William "Willie" Overton
Great-grandfather

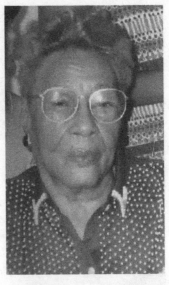

Geraldine Overton
"Momma Gearl" Great-
grandmother

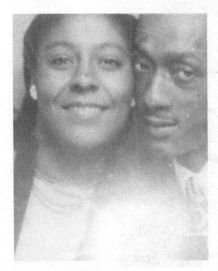

Aunty Mary and
Uncle Frederick (Booster)
Overton

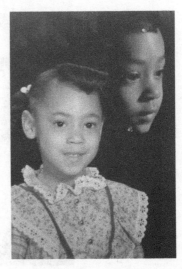

Ernestine Ford -
sister

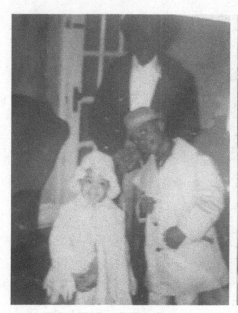
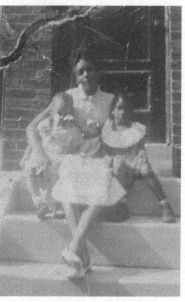

James (Jof) and Tina
Easter morning in 1978

Rosalee Ford Grandmother
(mother's mother) with
2 of her children
William" Sonny", and
Ernestine "Tina"

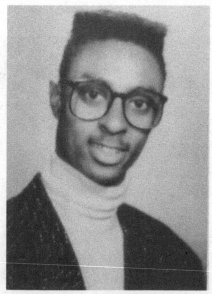

James Ford (Jasmine)
High School Graduation pic
in 1990

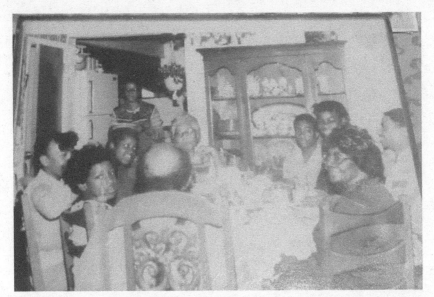

Clockwise starting from bottom front: William Overton (Great-grandfather), Opio (2nd Cousin), Terrell (1st cousin and daughter of my Aunt Tina), Sister of Opio, coming out of the kitchen is Great Aunt Desiree, Geraldine "Momma Geral" Overton, Dondie (1st cousin and brother of Terrell), Katrinka (1st cousin and daughter of Aunt Alease"Lisa", Tony (2nd cousin) and Alease " Fordie" Ford (Great- grandmother)

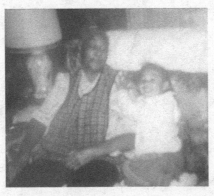

Aunt Mary and my niece
Ariana

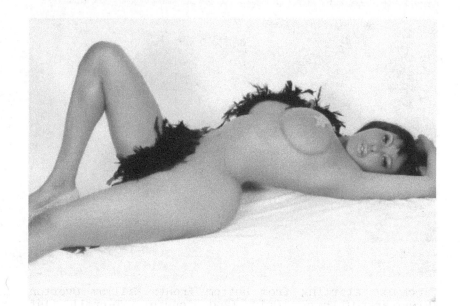

cover of adult magazine where I was recognized
as National TS escort of the year
and advertisement photo in 2006

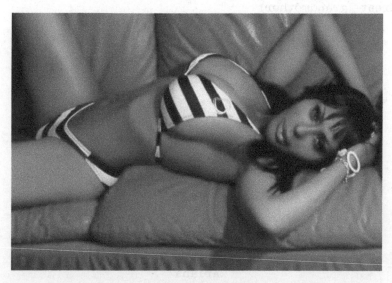

escort advertisements photo in 2007

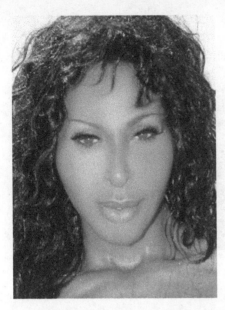

escort advertisement

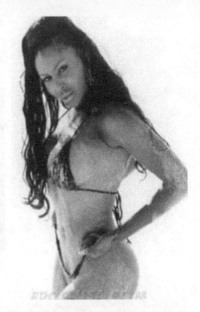

escort advertisement
photo from 2003 to 2015

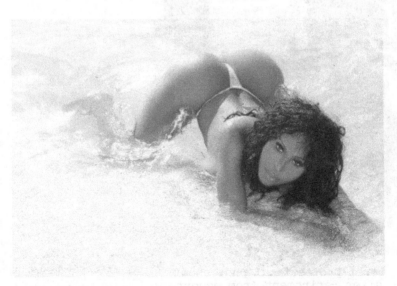

escort advertisement from 2010 to 2017

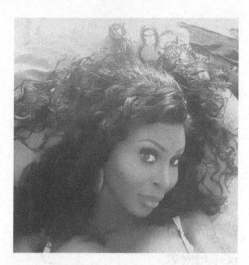

escort advertisement

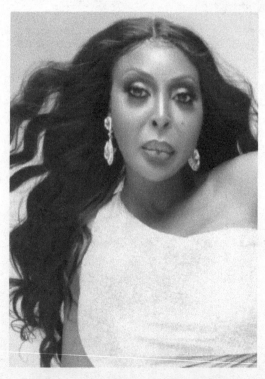

first professional photoshoot
after retirement from escort
business. Photo taken in summer of
2020 at the age of 48 years old.

300

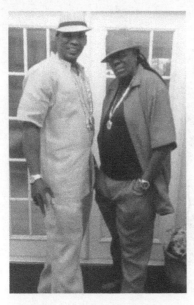 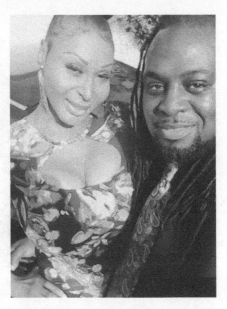

Members of the clan.
(L) Pic of Renee (trans
brother of Raquel), and
(R) Quinn Quinn

Pic of me and Cedric in the
parking lot of New Birth
Baptist Church in Miami
in 2014

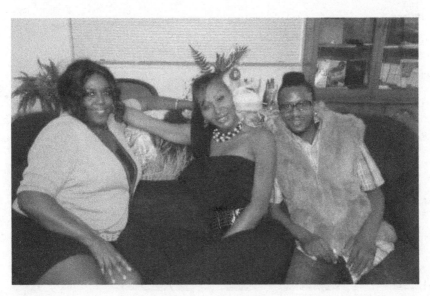

photo of the clan- Raquel, me and Diego at Thanksgiving
dinner at Mrs. Loretta's in 2014

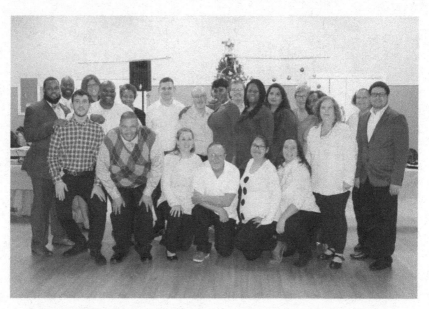

Giving back to the clients we serve and love at our
annual Client Gala in December 2018.

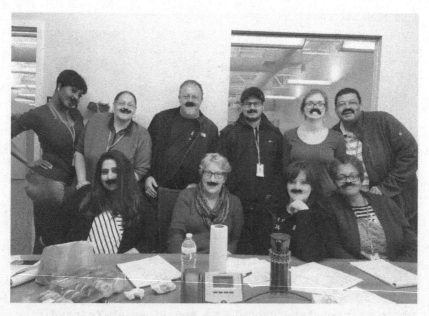

FAHASS staff pose in mustaches
after a Care Services Program meeting in 2017.

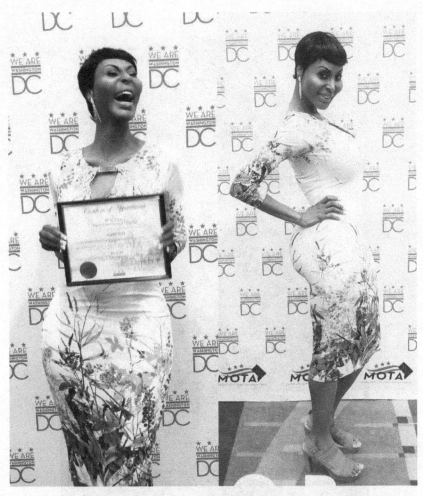

Swearing in Ceremony of the Washington DC Regional
Planning Commission on Health and HIV on May 31, 2018.

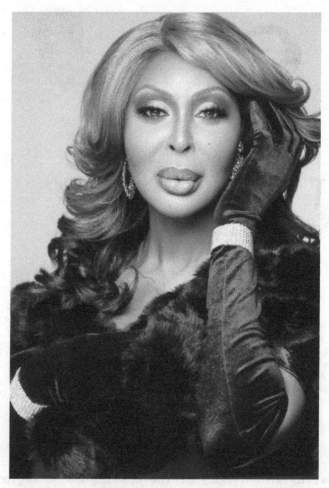

Pic of Jasmine Christine Ford, Author

CPSIA information can be obtained
at www.ICGtesting.com
Printed in the USA
LVHW032334220621
690926LV00017B/345